UPDATED

METABOLIC CONFUSION DIET PLAN

For

ENDOMORPH WOMEN

Complete Guide With Delicious Endomorph Diet Recipes And 21 Days Meal Plan To Boost Metabolism And Lose Weight

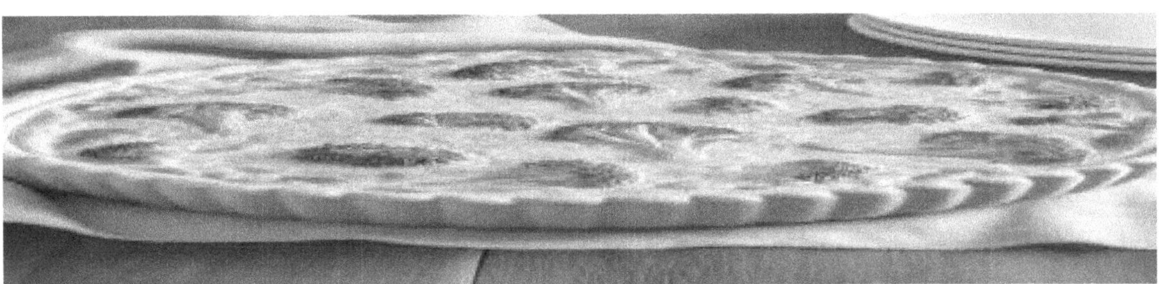

GRAHAM SCHMIDT

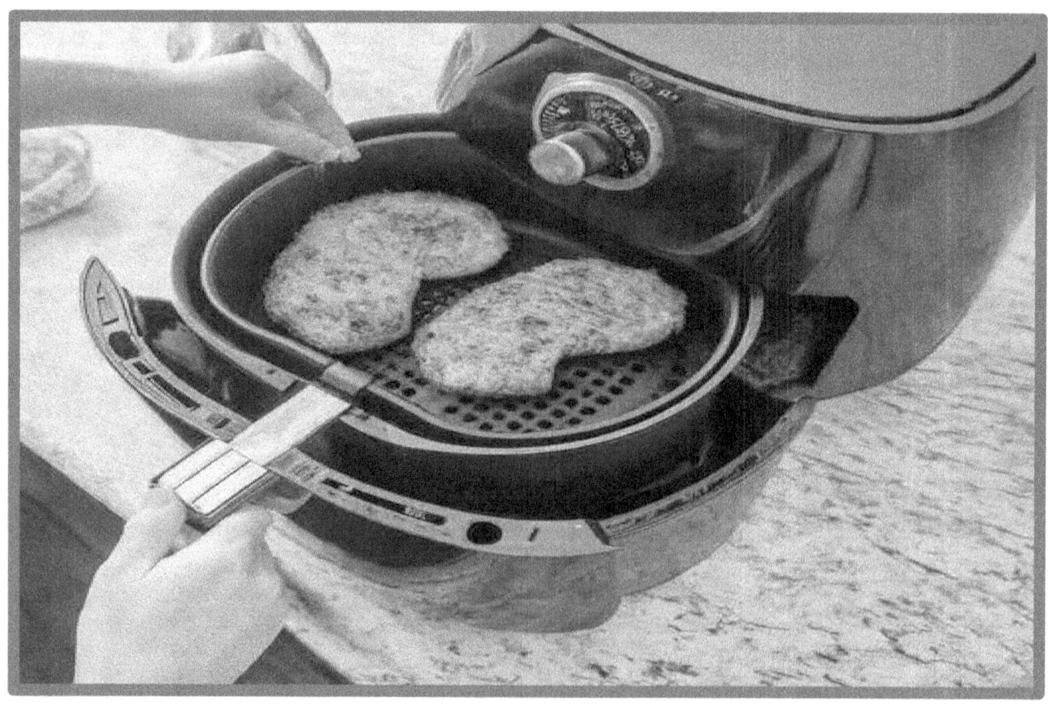

TABLE OF CONTENTS

INTRODUCTION

Tired of diets that leave you feeling hungry, restricted, and frustrated? Ready to ditch the endless cycle of weight loss and regain for a lifestyle that makes you feel strong, energized, and in control?

If you're an endomorph woman, you've likely been told that eating less and exercising more is the only way to reach your body goals. But what if there's a smarter way? A way to eat delicious, satisfying food, boost your metabolism and finally shed those stubborn pounds for good?

This cookbook is your solution.

My Mission, Your Transformation

I'm Graham Schmidt, and as a certified Nutritionist, I've dedicated my career to helping women just like you break free from diet dogma. After years of seeing endomorph women struggle, I realized there had to be a better way – an approach focused on nourishing your body, not punishing it. This cookbook isn't just about the food you eat. It's about empowering you to rewrite your relationship with food and transform your health in the process.

You're not doomed to struggle with your weight simply because of your body type. While endomorphs often have slower metabolisms, that doesn't mean you can't achieve your goals. This book will dismantle those myths and show you how simple dietary strategies, combined with the right exercise, can unlock your body's natural fat-burning potential.

Forget about chasing someone else's definition of "ideal." True success is feeling confident in your own skin and fueled by a diet that nourishes you, not depletes you. This cookbook will show you how to ditch restrictive eating, embrace delicious, satisfying meals, and finally take control of your health journey.

Are you ready for a change, a transformation that sticks? Then let's begin!

Let me know your thoughts. We can adjust the tone, level of science-focused language, and anything else to make it perfect for your vision!

CHAPTER ONE

The Endomorph Myth: Bust Common Misconceptions About Endomorph Bodies And Metabolism

If you identify as an endomorph, chances are you've been bombarded with information—some helpful, some downright harmful—about your body type. You've likely heard about the struggles with stubborn weight, the constant battle against a sluggish metabolism, and the frustration that comes with yo-yo dieting. It's no wonder many endomorph women feel defeated before they even begin their health journeys.

But what if I told you a lot of what you believe about your endomorph body is just plain wrong? That's right, it's time to dismantle those myths and misconceptions, and empower you with the knowledge to finally make lasting changes.

What is an Endomorph, Really?

Let's start with the basics. Body type classifications, including endomorphs, come from a theory developed in the 1940s. While there are some general characteristics associated with endomorphs—like a softer, rounder physique and a tendency to gain weight more easily—there's immense diversity within these categories.

The truth is, everyone's body is unique. Genetics, lifestyle, and countless other factors influence how you store fat, build muscle, and respond to diet and exercise. Blaming your body type for any struggles is an oversimplification that does way more harm than good.

Debunking the Endomorph Diet Trap

Here are some of the most common myths endomorph women are bombarded with, and why they hold no truth:

Myth #1: Endomorphs Are Destined to be Overweight

While endomorphs might be predisposed to storing fat more easily and may have a naturally slower metabolism, it doesn't mean they're destined to carry excess weight. With the right nutrition and exercise plan, anyone, regardless of body type, can achieve a healthy weight and lean, strong body.

Myth #2: Endomorphs Need Drastic Calorie Restriction to Lose Weight

Starving yourself is never the answer. Extreme dieting can actually backfire! It disrupts hormones, messes with your metabolism, and leads to unhealthy cravings and bingeing. A balanced approach emphasizing whole foods, protein, and healthy fats is the key to sustainable weight loss and optimal health.

Myth #3: Excessive Cardio is the Only Way for Endomorphs to Burn Calories

While cardio plays a role in fitness, strength training is your best friend. Building muscle increases metabolic rate, meaning your body burns more calories even at rest. Don't fear getting "bulky," ladies! You'll gain a toned and defined physique as you improve your body composition.

Myth #4: You Can't Change Your Body Type

Your genes certainly influence your shape and tendencies, but they're not your destiny. Through consistent healthy habits, you can change your body composition—meaning more muscle, less body fat. This translates into a metabolism that functions more efficiently, aiding in your wellness efforts.

Ditch the one-size-fits-all approach that so often leaves endomorph women feeling frustrated. Your individual needs and goals matter! Here's the key: understanding how your body works, learning to fuel it properly, and discovering fitness strategies that empower you to reach your full potential.

Rather than fighting against your body type, it's time to harness its strengths. Endomorphs often respond incredibly well to strength training and find immense satisfaction in building strength. It's a win-win: boosted metabolism, sculpted physique, and sky-high confidence.

The Bottom Line:

Forget those limitations placed on you by the "endomorph" label. You have boundless potential within you. This cookbook is a tool to unlock that potential, ditch diet myths, and find a truly empowering approach to health and wellness.

CHAPTER TWO

Beyond Metabolic Confusion

The phrase "metabolic confusion" has become a huge buzzword in the diet industry. Unfortunately, it's often surrounded by exaggerated claims, misinformation, and potentially harmful practices. Let's clear things up and understand how this concept can be leveraged in a safe and sustainable way.

The Truth About Our Metabolism

Your metabolism isn't a static number; it's a complex system that constantly adapts to changing circumstances. When you consistently restrict calories, your body responds by slowing your metabolism to conserve energy. It's your body protecting you from what it perceives as a lack of resources. While this helps explain why the initial weight loss of restrictive diets often plateaus, this doesn't mean your metabolism is broken!

The idea behind metabolic confusion is to introduce variety to prevent your body from fully adapting to a calorie deficit. However, extreme calorie zig-zagging or prolonged periods of severe restriction aren't the solution. They can disrupt hormone levels, make weight maintenance harder, lead to loss of lean muscle, and create an unhealthy relationship with food.

The Balanced Approach: Sustainable Cycling vs. Extreme Dieting

This cookbook takes a different approach, focusing on a sustainable model of calorie cycling. Let's break down why it's superior to drastic approaches:

Protecting Your Metabolism: Periods of moderate calorie restriction are necessary for weight loss but going too extreme can harm your metabolic rate. Planned higher-calorie days signal to your body there's no food shortage and help maintain a healthier metabolism.

Muscle Power: When calories get too low, you lose more than just fat. Your body may break down precious muscle for energy, negatively impacting your metabolic rate long-term. Sustaining lean muscle mass is vital for fat burning!

Fighting Cravings and Binges: Extreme diets are a recipe for bingeing. Strategic higher-calorie days help regulate hunger hormones and keep your willpower strong, preventing diet-wrecking slip-ups.

Focus on the Long-Term: It's about far more than a number on the scale. Balanced nutrition and flexible eating habits create lasting changes for whole-body wellness, promoting mental and physical health.

Quality Over Quantity: The Importance of Food Choices

Calorie cycling isn't a free-for-all! It's still about fueling your body with quality food. While there's room for flexibility, those extra calories on higher-intake days will largely come from whole, nutrient-dense sources, not empty-calorie treats.

The Power of Combining Strategies

A low-carb, high-protein approach is a powerful ally in managing your weight and promoting healthy metabolic function. This style of eating naturally helps control hunger, stabilize blood sugar levels, and preserve lean muscle mass.

By combining this nutritional focus with planned calorie cycling days, you create an effective strategy to boost your metabolism, promote healthy fat burning, and prevent long-term metabolic slowdown. Additionally, the occasional higher-carb allowance that comes with cycling can improve overall mood, energy levels, and dietary adherence in the long run.

In the next chapter, we'll discuss why a low-carb, high-protein approach is an optimal foundation for weight management and how this strategy works perfectly hand-in-hand with sustainable calorie cycling.

Low-Carb, High-Protein Power

You may be wary of a diet plan that allows you to consume a lot of protein and healthy fats while limiting starchy foods if you've previously had trouble losing weight. We've been taught that fat is harmful and that carbohydrates are necessary for energy, after all.

Time to reconsider those out-of-date notions! An increasing amount of studies demonstrates that a high-protein, low-carb diet might be revolutionary, particularly for endomorph women. Now let's dissect the research and reveal the potent advantages of this strategy.

Low-carb, high-protein diets are very popular, although their exact definition is still up for debate among clinicians.

One of two classifications for a high-protein, low-carb diet is typically used by experts:

- Through the measurement of an individual's daily "carbohydrate load."
- By figuring out how much protein and fat—two other macronutrients—are consumed in relation to the percentage of carbohydrates consumed.

For people who are not following a diet, the typical suggested daily allowance is 45 to 65 percent of their meals. A person on a low-carb diet may consume:

- fewer than 10% of their calories from carbohydrates (a very low-carb diet)
- a low-carb diet that contains more than 26% carbs
- a diet with a reasonable amount of carbohydrates, between 26 and 44 percent.

You'll need to eat more fat or protein to make up for the energy you lose when you consume fewer carbohydrates. One diet that lowers carbohydrates and raises fats is the ketogenic diet; a typical "keto" diet consists of 70% fat, 20% protein, and 10% carbohydrates.

A diet heavy in protein is the alternative. For adults, the recommended amount of protein on a regular diet is about 8 grams per kilogram of body weight (a little higher for those who exercise regularly or have an extremely active lifestyle). You might have more if you eat a high-protein diet.

Advantages of a Low-Carb, High-Protein Diet

The most significant benefit of a high-protein, low-carb diet is its ability to promote weight loss, particularly in individuals who are obese or overweight.

Studies show that low-carb diets are exceptionally successful in optimizing weight reduction throughout the first six to twelve months of the program. There is conflicting evidence on the relationship between eating a lot of protein and losing weight, but one study found that dieters who increased their protein intake also lost more weight than those who did not.

Apart from losing weight, the low-carb, high-protein diet may offer:

- Enhanced muscle repair: Since protein is essential for both muscle growth and repair, a high-protein, low-carb diet may be a great option if you're trying to lose weight and improve your fitness.

- Greater satiety — People who consume diets high in carbohydrates frequently experience spikes and falls in blood sugar, which can lead to overeating at meal times. Diets high in protein can increase satiety levels and reduce overindulgence tendencies in many individuals.

- More stable blood sugar: Whether or not you have been diagnosed with diabetes or insulin resistance, it's crucial to maintain a balanced blood glucose level. Your body will have a consistent supply of fuel if your blood sugar is stable, which reduces the likelihood of energy "crashes" over the day.

Low-Carb, High-Protein Diets and Ketosis: What's the Connection?

The term "ketosis" is probably familiar to you if you've been researching low-carb diets. A metabolic state known as ketosis may occur if you have severely reduced your intake of carbohydrates. Your body uses ketones—which are produced by your liver when it draws on fat reserves—as a fuel source when it stops using carbs, or sugars.

- Liver and renal problems: The correct breakdown of the food you eat depends on your kidneys and liver. Because proteins and fats are harder to digest than carbohydrates, some ketogenic diets can make them overworked or worsen pre-existing conditions.

- Prolonged digestion Diets high in fat may cause constipation and delayed digestion. Since the body gets most of its fiber from diets high in carbohydrates, cutting these foods may make it harder to produce regular bowel movements.

Finally, it may be challenging to get the vitamins and minerals found in complex natural carbs like whole produce if you drastically cut your overall carbohydrate consumption through low-carb meals. In order to make sure you can fulfill all of your nutritional needs, make sure you research the benefits and drawbacks of the keto diet and speak with a healthcare professional before attempting any version of it.

Who Should Try a Low-Carb, High-Protein Diet

Low-carb, high-protein diets might be more beneficial for some persons than for others. Usually, medical professionals advise this dietary strategy for:

- People who are overweight or obese
- People who are at risk of developing metabolic syndrome
- Individuals who are insulin resistant or who may become so in the future
- People with type 2 diabetes

Low-carb diets are a crucial component of a diabetic's treatment regimen. People with diabetes may also reduce their chance of consuming trans and saturated fats, which can be detrimental to their health, by emphasizing high protein intake rather than high fat intake.

Drawbacks To A Low-Carb, High-Protein Diet

Low-carb, high-protein diets don't appear to be harmful to your health at this time, at least not without solid evidence. While some studies have suggested that certain people may be more susceptible to cardiovascular disease when following a low-carb diet, no clear correlation has been found.

Therefore, before beginning this diet if you're trying to lose weight, keep the following things in mind:

- Kidney health: Before beginning any high-protein diet, speak with your doctor if you have ever experienced kidney disease or damage. Regularly consuming high protein diets might strain the kidneys and increase the risk of kidney stones.
- Nutrition over the long term: Low-carb diets are typically advised as a temporary strategy for individuals seeking to achieve a healthy target weight. These are not intended to be a lifelong way of eating, unless you have diabetes or have been specifically instructed to do so by a healthcare professional.
- Convenience: Because measuring macronutrients is a lot of work, low-carb, high-protein diets may not be feasible for certain people. Nevertheless, adopting a low-carb, high-protein diet might be lot easier than you might imagine if you collaborate with your doctor and a dietitian.

CHAPTER THREE

The Art of Nutrient Cycling

If the idea of sticking to a low-carb plan every single day feels daunting, there's good news! Nutrient cycling is the key to making this approach not only enjoyable but incredibly effective. Think of it as a strategic way to give your body the boost it needs while preventing plateaus and keeping you motivated.

Why Cycling Works

The term "metabolic confusion" gets thrown around a lot, but it often leads to misconceptions. Our approach isn't about drastically fluctuating calories or throwing your body into chaos. Instead, it's a carefully planned method to optimize your metabolism and support continued progress.

Here's how nutrient cycling works in your favor:

Prevents Metabolic Slowdown: When you're consistently in a calorie deficit, your body can adapt by slowing your metabolism to conserve energy. Planned higher-carb days help signal that there's no food shortage, preserving your metabolic rate.

Hormone Balance: Cycling your intake supports hormones like leptin, which helps regulate hunger and energy expenditure. This can prevent cravings and keep you feeling satisfied.

Boost Workout Performance: Strategic carb intake before a tough workout can give you energy and help you maximize your training sessions.

Psychological Break: Let's face it, even the most dedicated plan can feel restrictive. Higher-carb days offer a well-timed mental break, making it easier to stick with your plan in the long run.

Finding Your Rhythm: Cycling Strategies

There's no one-size-fits-all approach. Here are a few common examples to get you started:

- **The Classic: 2:1 Cycle**
    - Two low-carb, high-protein days.
    - One moderate-to-high carb day.
    - Repeat this pattern throughout the week.

- **The Weekend Recharge: 5:2 Cycle**
    - o Five low-carb, high-protein days.
    - o Two moderate-carb days, often placed on the weekend for flexibility.
- **Active Days: Adjust Based on Training**
    - o Low-carb on rest days or light workout days.
    - o Include more carbs on days with intense workouts.

Important Note: Even on higher-carb days, prioritize whole foods! Think sweet potatoes, fruit, whole grains, and legumes, rather than processed junk foods.

Tips for Success

- **Track and Tweak:** Start with one of the example strategies. Pay attention to your energy, hunger, and workouts. Adjust your carb intake and the timing of cycle days as needed.
- **Listen to Your Body:** There are no hard rules. Experiment to find what works for you. If you're feeling constantly sluggish or find yourself craving carbs, adjust those higher-carb days.
- **Focus on Progress, Not Perfection:** Slip-ups happen! Don't get discouraged, keep focusing on the big picture and building sustainable habits.

CHAPTER FOUR

The Delicious Details

Endomorph-Friendly Ingredients: Your Delicious Toolkit

This chapter isn't just a grocery list; it's about understanding *why* these foods are your allies for weight loss, improved insulin sensitivity, and overall health. Let's break it down into categories, emphasizing their unique benefits while keeping things exciting! As shown in the table below:

Food Lists	Summary
Protein Powerhouses: Your Metabolic Boosters	
Lean Meats & Poultry	Chicken breast, turkey breast, lean cuts of beef, pork tenderloin, and ground options (90% lean or higher). High in protein, iron, and B vitamins – essential for muscle building and energy.
Seafood	Salmon, tuna, cod, shrimp, sardines – packed with protein and omega-3 fatty acids, promoting heart health and reducing inflammation.
Eggs	Nature's perfect food! Versatile, affordable protein, plus healthy fats and essential nutrients.
Plant-Based Options	Tofu, tempeh, lentils, beans, edamame – excellent choices for vegetarians or for adding variety to your protein sources.
Vegetable Superstars: Low in Carbs, High in Nutrients	
Leafy Greens	Spinach, kale, Swiss chard, arugula – packed with fiber, vitamins, and minerals

	that support blood sugar control and overall health. Cruciferous Crew: Broccoli, cauliflower, Brussels sprouts, cabbage – fiber-rich and promote detoxification, particularly beneficial for hormone balance.
Other Low-Carb Veggies	Asparagus, bell peppers, mushrooms, zucchini, green beans – add flavor, essential nutrients, and keep you feeling full.
Healthy Fats: For Flavor and Satisfaction	
Avocados	Creamy, delicious, and full of fiber and heart-healthy monounsaturated fats. Help stabilize blood sugar and boost satiety levels.
Nuts and Seeds	Almonds, walnuts, pecans, chia seeds, pumpkin seeds – sources of protein, fiber, essential minerals, and antioxidants. Perfect for snacking!
Olive Oil and Coconut Oil	Heart-healthy cooking fats and sources of energy. Coconut oil has shown potential to boost metabolism slightly.

Foods to Limit or Avoid

- **Processed Meats:** Most bacon, sausage, deli meats – contain harmful fats, nitrates, and added sugars. Look for minimally processed options, or lean cuts cooked at home.
- **Refined Grains & Sugars:** White bread/pasta, pastries, chips, candy, juices, sugary drinks – spike blood sugar, promote cravings, and nutrient-poor.

- **"Diet" Foods:** Many low-fat or sugar-free products are packed with artificial ingredients that can disrupt the gut and metabolism.
- **Excessively Fatty Foods:** Deep-fried foods, overly cheesy dishes, heavy sauces – while a small amount of healthy fats is vital, too much can stall progress

CHAPTER FIVE

BREAKFASTS TO BOOST

CLOUD EGGS WITH SPINACH & FETA

Yields: 2 servings | **Prep Time:** 5 minutes | **Cook Time:** 12-15 minutes | **Total Time:** 17-20 minutes

INGREDIENTS

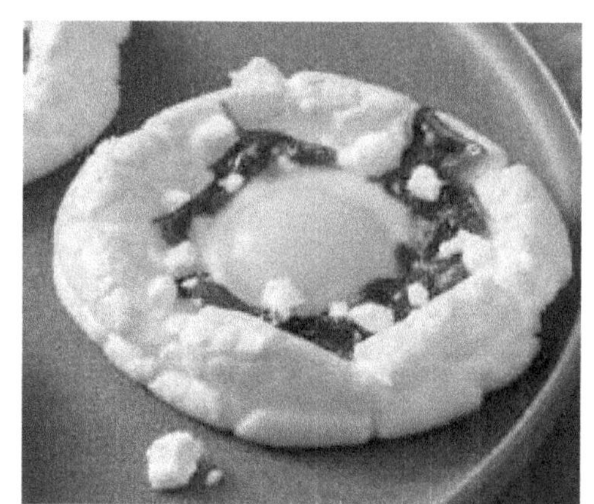

- 4 large egg whites
- 1/2 teaspoon cream of tartar
- 1/4 cup crumbled feta cheese
- 2 cups baby spinach
- 1 tablespoon olive oil
- Salt and black pepper to taste
- Fresh herbs for garnish (optional, such as chives or dill)

INSTRUCTIONS

1. Preheat oven to 450°F (230°C). Line a baking sheet with parchment paper.

2. In a large bowl, beat the egg whites and cream of tartar until stiff peaks form.

3. Gently fold in the feta cheese.

4. Heat the olive oil in a skillet over medium heat. Add the spinach and cook until wilted, about 2 minutes. Season with salt and pepper.

5. On the prepared baking sheet, create two large mounds of egg whites, leaving a slight indentation in the center of each.

6. Bake for 10-12 minutes, or until the egg whites are set and slightly golden.

7. Divide the wilted spinach between the two egg white nests.

8. Bake for an additional 2-3 minutes, or until the spinach is heated through.

9. Garnish with fresh herbs, if desired, and serve immediately.

TIPS

- For extra fluffy egg whites, make sure the bowl and beaters are very clean and free of grease.
- You can add a pinch of chili flakes for a little kick.
- Experiment with different fillings like mushrooms, tomatoes, or bacon.

NUTRITIONAL FACTS

- Calories: 150

- Protein: 15 g

- Fat: 10 g

- Carbohydrates: 4 g

- Fiber: 3 g

KETO FRITTATA WITH SAUSAGE & PEPPERS

Yields: 6 servings | **Prep Time:** 10 minutes | **Cook Time:** 30-35 minutes | **Total Time:** 40-45 minutes

INGREDIENTS

- 1 tablespoon olive oil
- 1/2 pound Italian sausage (spicy or sweet), casing removed
- 1/2 cup chopped onion
- 1/2 cup chopped green bell pepper
- 1/2 cup chopped red bell pepper
- 1/2 teaspoon salt
- 1/4 teaspoon black pepper
- 8 large eggs
- 1/4 cup heavy cream
- 1/2 cup shredded cheddar cheese

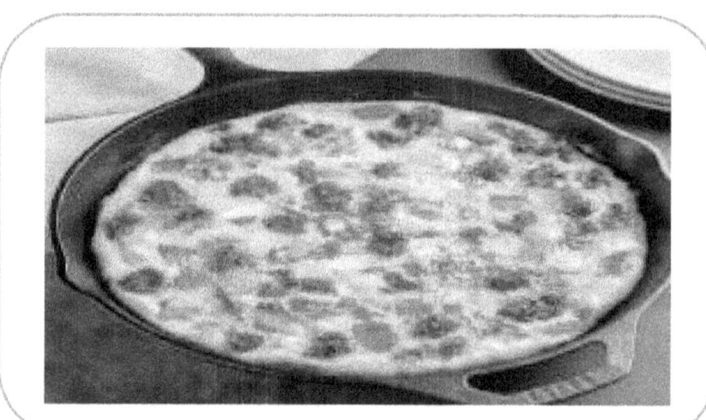

INSTRUCTIONS

1. Preheat oven to 375°F (190°C). Grease a 9-inch pie dish or cast-iron skillet.

2. Heat the olive oil in a large skillet over medium heat. Add the sausage and cook, breaking it up with a spoon, until browned, about 5 minutes.

3. Add the onion, green bell pepper, and red bell pepper to the skillet. Cook, stirring occasionally, until softened, about 5 minutes. Season with salt and pepper.

4. In a medium bowl, whisk together the eggs and heavy cream.

5. Pour the egg mixture into the prepared dish. Top with the sausage and pepper mixture, then sprinkle with the cheddar cheese.

6. Bake for 30-35 minutes, or until the eggs are set and the center is no longer jiggly. Let cool slightly before slicing and serving.

- For a vegetarian version, swap the sausage for crumbled firm tofu or add an extra cup of chopped vegetables.
- Spice things up with a pinch of red pepper flakes or your favorite hot sauce.
- Leftovers can be stored in the refrigerator for up to 3 days. Reheat slices in the microwave or toaster oven.

NUTRITIONAL FACTS

- Calories: 240

- Protein: 18 g

- Fat: 18 g

- Total Carbohydrates: 3 g

- Net Carbohydrates: 2 g

- Fiber: 1 g

CRUSTLESS BROCCOLI & CHEDDAR QUICHE

Yields: 6 servings | **Prep Time:** 15 minutes | **Cook Time:** 35-40 minutes | **Total Time:** 50-55 minutes

INGREDIENTS

- 1 tablespoon olive oil
- 1 cup chopped onion
- 2 cups chopped broccoli florets
- 1/2 teaspoon salt
- 1/4 teaspoon black pepper
- 8 large eggs
- 1/2 cup heavy cream
- 1cup shredded cheddar cheese

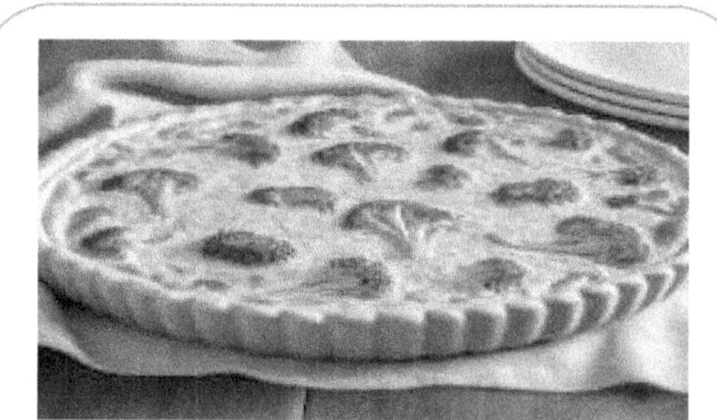

INSTRUCTIONS

1. Preheat oven to 375°F (190°C). Grease a 9-inch pie dish or cast-iron skillet.

2. Heat the olive oil in a large skillet over medium heat. Add the onion and cook until softened, about 5 minutes.

3. Add the broccoli florets, salt, and pepper to the skillet. Cook, stirring occasionally, until the broccoli is tender-crisp, about 5 minutes.

4. In a medium bowl, whisk together the eggs and heavy cream.

5. Stir in half of the cheddar cheese into the egg mixture.

6. Spread the broccoli and onion mixture evenly in the prepared dish. Pour the egg mixture over top. Sprinkle with the remaining cheddar cheese.

7. Bake for 35-40 minutes, or until the eggs are set and the center is no longer jiggly. Let cool slightly before slicing and serving.

- Add other vegetables: Mushrooms, spinach, or chopped bell peppers would work well.

- Get creative with cheese: Try Swiss, Gruyere, or a blend of cheeses for different flavors.

- Make-ahead meal: Assemble the quiche the night before and bake it in the morning for a hassle-free breakfast.

NUTRITIONAL FACTS

- Calories: 220

- Protein: 15 g

- Fat: 16 g

- Total Carbohydrates: 5 g

- Net Carbohydrates: 3g

- Fiber: 2g

BAKED EGGS IN AVOCADO

Yields: 2 servings | **Prep Time:** 5 minutes | **Cook Time:** 15-20 minutes | **Total Time:** 20-25 minutes

INGREDIENTS

- 2 large avocados, halved and pitted
- 4 large eggs
- Salt and black pepper to taste
- Optional toppings: chopped fresh herbs (chives, parsley, dill), hot sauce, crumbled bacon, shredded cheese

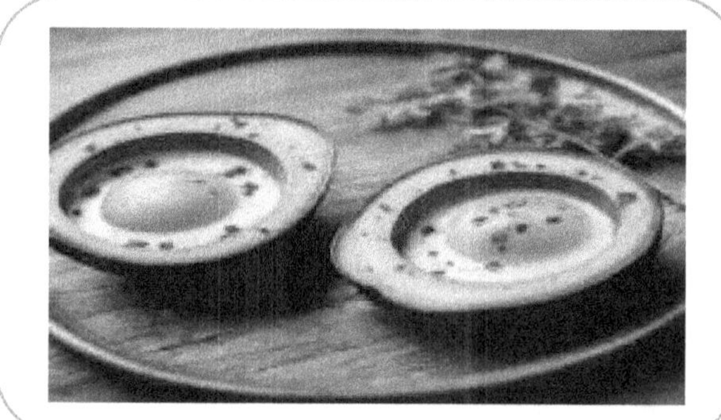

INSTRUCTIONS

1. Preheat oven to 425°F (220°C).

2. Place the avocado halves, cut-side up, in a baking dish. If needed, gently scoop out a bit of extra avocado flesh from the center to widen the hole for the egg.

3. Crack one egg into each avocado half. Season with salt and pepper to taste.

4. Bake for 15-20 minutes, or until the egg whites are set and the yolks are still slightly runny (adjust time for your desired doneness).

5. Top with desired toppings like fresh herbs, hot sauce, crumbled bacon, or shredded cheese. Serve immediately.

TIPS

- To keep the avocados from wobbling, use a muffin tin or nestle them in crumpled aluminum foil in a baking dish.
- For extra richness, add a dollop of sour cream or a sprinkle of crumbled feta cheese before serving.
- Let your imagination run wild with toppings: try chopped tomatoes, salsa, or a drizzle of pesto for variations.

NUTRITIONAL FACTS

- Calories: 250
- Protein: 14 g
- Fat: 22 g
- Total Carbohydrates: 7 g
- Net Carbohydrates: 4 g
- Fiber: 3 g

SHAKSHUKA-INSPIRED SCRAMBLE

Yields: 2 servings | **Prep Time:** 10 minutes | **Cook Time:** 15-20 minutes | **Total Time:** 25-30 minutes

INGREDIENTS

- 1 tablespoon olive oil
- 1/2 cup chopped onion
- 1/2 cup chopped green bell pepper
- 1/2 cup chopped red bell pepper
- 1 (14.5 ounce) can diced tomatoes, undrained
- 1/2 teaspoon cumin
- 1/4 teaspoon smoked paprika
- 1/4 teaspoon salt
- 1/8 teaspoon black pepper
- Pinch of red pepper flakes (optional, for heat)
- 4 large eggs
- Optional toppings: crumbled feta cheese, chopped fresh cilantro, avocado slices

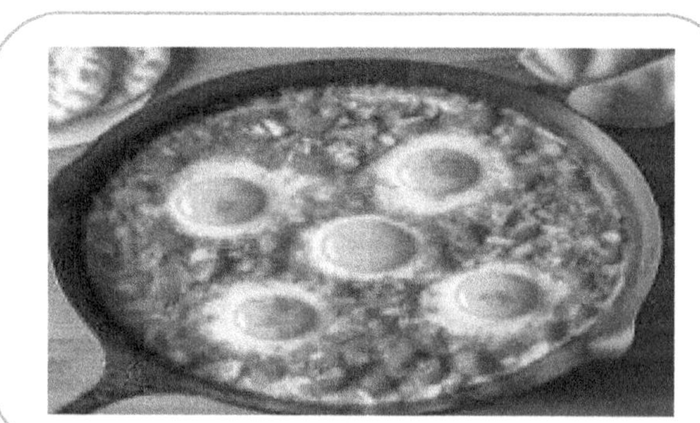

INSTRUCTIONS

1. Heat the olive oil in a large skillet over medium heat. Add the onion, green bell pepper, and red bell pepper. Cook, stirring occasionally, until softened, about 5 minutes.

2. Stir in the diced tomatoes, cumin, paprika, salt, pepper, and red pepper flakes (if using). Bring to a simmer and cook for 5 minutes, or until the sauce has thickened slightly.

3. Create four small wells in the tomato sauce. Crack one egg into each well.

4. Reduce heat to low, cover the skillet, and cook until the egg whites are set and the yolks are still runny, about 5-8 minutes (adjust for your desired doneness).

5. Top with desired toppings like crumbled feta cheese, chopped cilantro, or avocado slices. Serve immediately with your favorite low-carb bread or a side salad.

TIPS

- Spice it up: Experiment with different spice blends like harissa or za'atar for varied flavors.
- Add more protein: Stir in cooked ground sausage, crumbled chorizo, or shredded chicken for an even heartier scramble.
- Meal prep: Make a larger batch of the tomato sauce in advance and reheat for quick individual scrambles throughout the week.

NUTRITIONAL FACTS

- Calories: 320
- Protein: 18 g
- Fat: 22 g
- Total Carbohydrates: 16 g
- Net Carbohydrates: 12 g
- Fiber: 4 g

KETO EGG BITES

Yields: 12 egg bites **Prep Time:** 10 minutes **Cook Time:** 20-25 minutes **Total Time:** 30-35 minutes

INGREDIENTS

- 10 large eggs
- 1/2 cup heavy cream
- 1/2 teaspoon salt
- 1/4 teaspoon black pepper
- 1/2 cup shredded cheddar cheese

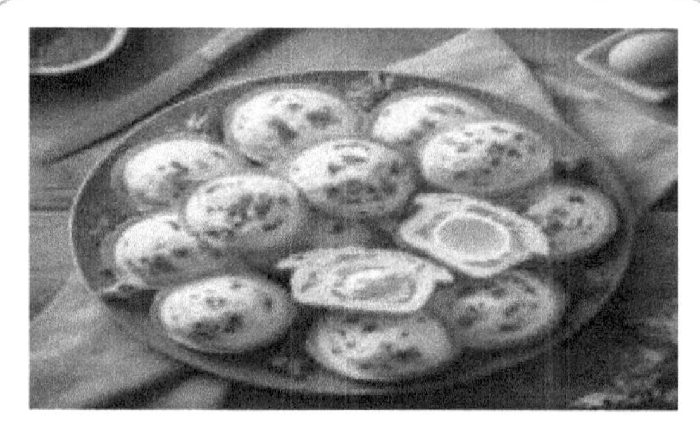

Mix-In Options (choose your favorite combos):

- **Spinach & Feta:** 1 cup chopped cooked spinach, 1/4 cup crumbled feta cheese
- **Bacon & Cheddar:** 1/2 cup cooked, crumbled bacon, 1/2 cup shredded cheddar cheese
- **Ham & Swiss:** 1/2 cup diced ham, 1/2 cup shredded Swiss cheese
- **Mushroom & Parmesan:** 1 cup sautéed mushrooms, 1/4 cup grated Parmesan cheese

INSTRUCTIONS

1. Preheat oven to 350°F (175°C). Grease a 12-cup muffin tin.

2. In a large bowl, whisk together the eggs, heavy cream, salt, and pepper.

3. Stir in the shredded cheddar cheese (for the base recipe).

4. Select your desired mix-in combination and add those ingredients to the egg mixture.

5. Divide the egg mixture evenly among the muffin cups.

6. Bake for 20-25 minutes, or until the egg bites are set and puffed up. Let cool slightly in the pan before removing.

TIPS

- Get creative with add-ins: Use your favorite vegetables, cheeses, or cooked meats.
- Prevent sticking: For easy removal, line muffin cups with parchment paper or silicone liners.
- Make-ahead & Storage: Egg bites are perfect for meal prep. Store leftovers in the refrigerator for up to 4 days or freeze for later.

NUTRITIONAL FACTS

- Calories: 80
- Protein: 6 g
- Fat: 6 g
- Total Carbohydrates: 1 g
- Net Carbohydrates: 1 g
- Fiber: 0 g

SCRAMBLED EGGS WITH SMOKED SALMON & DILL

Yields: 2 servings **Prep Time:** 5 minutes **Cook Time:** 5-7 minutes **Total Time:** 10-12 minutes

INGREDIENTS

- 1 tablespoon butter
- 4 large eggs
- 1/4 cup heavy cream or milk
- 1/2 teaspoon salt
- 1/4 teaspoon black pepper
- 3 ounces thinly sliced smoked salmon, chopped
- 2 tablespoons chopped fresh dill

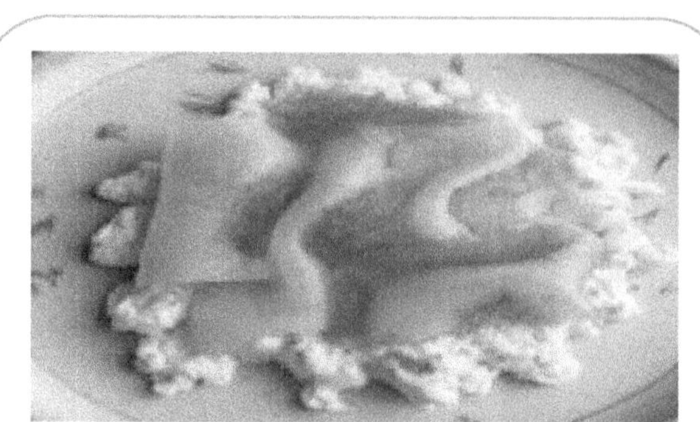

INSTRUCTIONS

1. Melt the butter in a medium nonstick skillet over medium heat.

2. In a small bowl, whisk together the eggs, heavy cream (or milk), salt, and pepper.

3. Pour the egg mixture into the skillet and cook, stirring gently, until the eggs are softly scrambled, about 3-5 minutes.

4. Gently fold in the smoked salmon and dill. Cook for an additional minute, just to warm through.

5. Serve immediately with your favorite low-carb sides, if desired.

TIPS

- Don't overcook: The eggs should be cooked through but still soft and creamy. Remove them from the heat just before they seem completely set.
- Cream Variations: Use sour cream or crème fraîche for extra richness.
- Other Herbs: Feel free to substitute your favorite fresh herbs like chives or tarragon.

NUTRITIONAL FACTS

- Calories: 300
- Protein: 22 g
- Fat: 24g
- Total Carbohydrates: 2 g
- Net Carbohydrates: 1g
- Fiber: 1 g

Yields: 2 wraps | **Prep Time:** 5 minutes | **Cook Time:** 5 minutes | **Total Time:** 10 minutes

INGREDIENTS

- 4 large eggs
- Salt and black pepper to taste
- 1 tablespoon butter or olive oil
- Fillings of your choice

Filling Suggestions:

- **Cream Cheese & Smoked Salmon**: Spread cream cheese on the egg wrap, top with smoked salmon, thinly sliced red onion, and capers.
- **Avocado & Turkey**: Layer slices of turkey breast, avocado, spinach, and a drizzle of hot sauce.
- **Ham & Swiss:** Thin slices of ham, Swiss cheese, and a smear of Dijon mustard.
- **Spinach & Feta:** Sautéed spinach with crumbled feta cheese and a sprinkle of red pepper flakes.

INSTRUCTIONS

1. In a small bowl, whisk together the eggs, salt, and pepper.

2. Heat a medium nonstick skillet over medium heat. Add the butter or olive oil.

3. Pour half of the egg mixture into the skillet and swirl to create a thin, even layer (similar to making crepes).

4. Cook until the underside is set and the top is mostly set, about 1-2 minutes. Flip and cook briefly on the other side.

5. Transfer the egg wrap to a plate. Repeat with the remaining egg mixture to make a second wrap.

6. Fill the egg wraps with your desired fillings and roll them up. Serve immediately.

- Thin is in: The thinner the egg layer, the easier it is to roll.

- Use a flexible spatula: This helps lift the delicate egg wraps from the pan.

- Warm fillings: For best results, use warm or room temperature fillings to prevent the egg wraps from cooling down too quickly.

NUTRITIONAL FACTS

Calories: 120

Protein: 10 g

Fat: 9 g

Total Carbohydrates: 1 g

Net Carbohydrates: 1 g

Fiber: 0 g

PROTEIN "FLUFF"

Yields: 1 serving **Prep Time:** 5 minutes **Total Time:** 5 minutes

INGREDIENTS

- 1 cup plain nonfat Greek yogurt
- 1 scoop low-carb protein powder (vanilla or flavor of your choice)
- 1/4 teaspoon sweetener of choice (optional - stevia, monk fruit, etc.)
- Optional: 1/4 teaspoon vanilla extract

INSTRUCTIONS

1. In a medium bowl, combine the Greek yogurt, protein powder, sweetener (if using), and vanilla extract (if using).

2. Using a hand mixer or a whisk, whip the mixture until it becomes light, fluffy, and doubled in volume. This will take about 2-3 minutes.

3. Serve immediately or chill in the refrigerator for a thicker texture.

- Flavor Variations: Experiment with different protein powder flavors (chocolate, strawberry, etc.) or add a pinch of cinnamon.
- Toppings: Top with fresh berries, a sprinkle of nuts or seeds, or a drizzle of sugar-free chocolate syrup for extra indulgence.
- Texture Tweaks: For a thicker fluff, use less yogurt or chill for longer. For a thinner consistency, add a splash of unsweetened almond milk.

NUTRITIONAL FACTS

- Calories: 180
- Protein: 35 g
- Fat: 1 g
- Total Carbohydrates: 8 g
- Net Carbohydrates: 7 g
- Fiber: 1 g

CAULIFLOWER "TOAST" WITH AVOCADO & SMOKED SALMON

Yields: 2 servings | **Prep Time:** 15 minutes | **Cook Time:** 20-25 minutes | **Total Time:** 35-40 minutes

INGREDIENTS

- 1/2 head cauliflower, cut into 1/2-inch thick slices
- 2 tablespoons olive oil
- 1/4 teaspoon salt
- 1/4 teaspoon black pepper
- 1 ripe avocado, mashed
- 4 ounces smoked salmon
- Optional toppings: a squeeze of lemon juice, capers, thinly sliced red onion, fresh dill

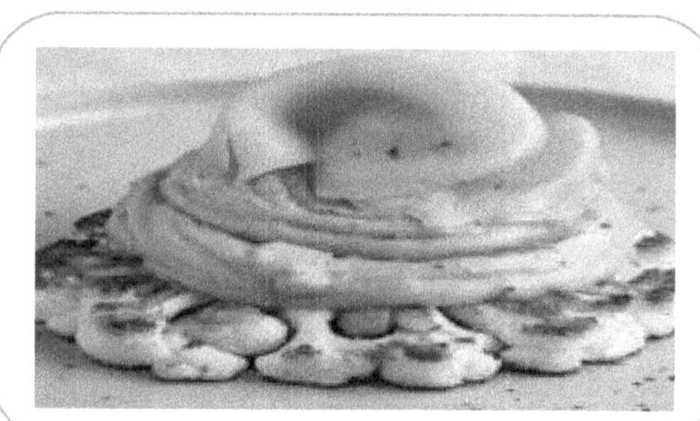

INSTRUCTIONS

1. **Preheat Oven:** Preheat oven to 425°F (220°C). Line a baking sheet with parchment paper.

2. **Prep Cauliflower "Toast":** Arrange the cauliflower slices on the prepared baking sheet. Brush both sides with olive oil and season with salt and pepper.

3. **Bake:** Bake for 20-25 minutes, or until tender and lightly browned, flipping halfway through.

4. **Assemble:** Spread mashed avocado on top of each cauliflower "toast." Layer with smoked salmon.

5. **Add Toppings:** Top with your desired additions like a squeeze of lemon juice, capers, dill, or thinly sliced red onion for extra flavor and crunch.

TIPS

- Keep it Thin: Cutting the cauliflower into thin slices is key for creating a sturdy "toast" base.
- Roasting vs. Pan-Frying: For a softer texture, you can pan-fry the cauliflower slices in olive oil instead of baking.
- Get Creative with Toppings: Try cream cheese and chives, a fried egg, or a dollop of pesto.

NUTRITIONAL FACTS

- Calories: 320

- Protein: 20 g

- Fat: 26 g

- Total Carbohydrates: 12 g

- Net Carbohydrates: 8 g

- Fiber: 4 g

PEANUT BUTTER PROTEIN SMOOTHIE

Yields: 1 serving **Prep Time:** 5 minutes **Blend Time:** 1 minute **Total Time:** 6 minutes

INGREDIENTS

- 1 cup unsweetened almond milk (or other low-carb milk alternative)
- 1 scoop low-carb vanilla protein powder
- 1/4 cup peanut butter (creamy or crunchy)
- 1/2 cup frozen spinach
- 1/2 cup ice cubes
- Optional: 1 tablespoon chia seeds or flaxseed for extra fiber
- Optional: A pinch of cinnamon for a flavor boost

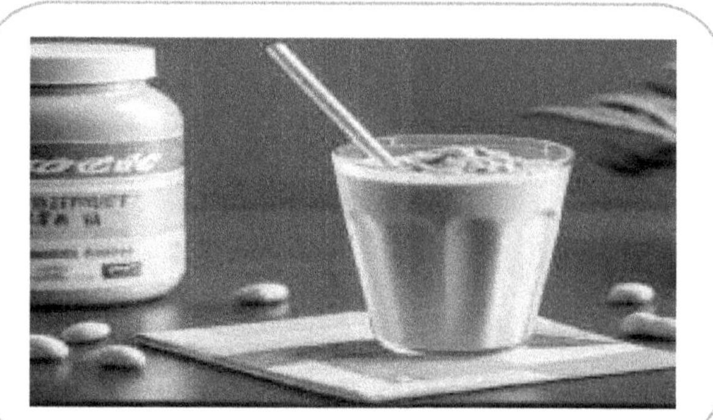

INSTRUCTIONS

1. Add all ingredients to a high-powered blender.

2. Blend until smooth and creamy. If it's too thick, add a splash more almond milk.

3. Pour into a glass and enjoy immediately.

- Customize Your Protein: Use your favorite low-carb protein powder. Chocolate would be delicious, too!
- Make it Ahead: Freeze individual smoothie packs with pre-portioned ingredients (minus the ice) for grab-and-go breakfasts.
- Greens Boost: Feel free to add other greens like kale or a handful of fresh mint.

NUTRITIONAL FACTS

- Calories: 350
- Protein: 30 g
- Fat: 20 g
- Total Carbohydrates: 22 g
- Net Carbohydrates: 16 g
- Fiber: 6 g

CHAPTER SIX

LUNCHTIME FUEL

SHRIMP & AVOCADO SALAD STUFFED PEPPERS

Yields: 4 servings | **Prep Time:** 15 minutes | **Cook Time:** 10 minutes | **Total Time:** 25 minutes

INGREDIENTS

- **1** pound medium shrimp, peeled and deveined
- 1 tablespoon olive oil
- 1/2 teaspoon salt
- 1/4 teaspoon black pepper
- 2 bell peppers (any color), halved and seeds removed
- 1 ripe avocado, mashed
- 1/4 cup chopped fresh cilantro or parsley
- 2 tablespoons lime juice
- 1/4 cup mayonnaise (or use plain Greek yogurt for lower fat)
- Hot sauce to taste (optional)

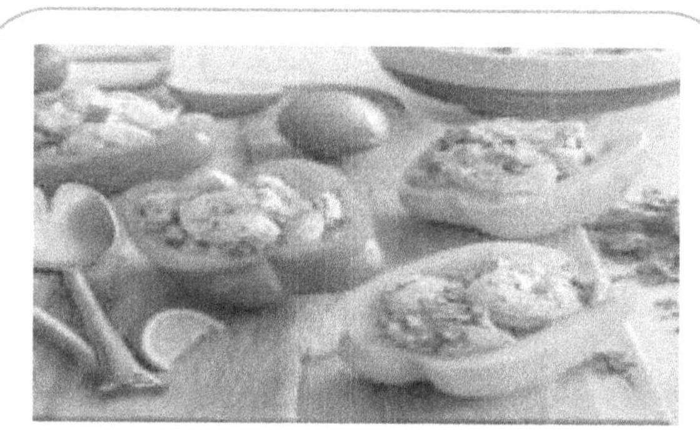

INSTRUCTIONS

1. **Cook the Shrimp:** Heat olive oil in a large skillet over medium-high heat. Add the shrimp, salt, and pepper. Cook, stirring occasionally, until pink and cooked through, about 3-5 minutes. Remove from pan and set aside.
2. **Prepare the Peppers:** While the shrimp cooks, prepare your bell pepper "bowls."
3. **Make the Salad:** In a medium bowl, combine mashed avocado, cilantro, lime juice, mayonnaise (or yogurt), and hot sauce (if using). Gently fold in cooled shrimp.

4. **Stuff & Serve:** Divide the shrimp and avocado salad evenly among the pepper halves. Serve immediately or chill for later.

- Grill the Peppers: For extra flavor, grill the pepper halves for a few minutes before stuffing for a touch of smoky char.
- Spice it Up: Add a pinch of chili powder or cayenne to the shrimp for a kick.
- Make it Ahead: Assemble the salad and stuff the peppers up to a day in advance. Store covered in the refrigerator.

NUTRITIONAL FACTS

Calories: 340

Protein: 28 g

Fat: 24 g

Total Carbohydrates: 14 g

Net Carbohydrates: 10 g

Fiber: 4 g

ZUCCHINI NOODLE SALAD WITH GRILLED CHICKEN

Yields: 4 servings | **Prep Time:** 15 minutes | **Cook Time:** 10-15 minutes | **Total Time:** 25-30 minutes

INGREDIENTS

- 1 pound boneless, skinless chicken breasts
- 1 tablespoon olive oil
- Salt and black pepper to taste
- 2 medium zucchini, spiralized
- 1 cup cherry tomatoes, halved
- 1/2 cup cucumber, diced
- 1/4 cup crumbled feta cheese (optional)

Vinaigrette:
- 3 tablespoons olive oil
- 2 tablespoons lemon juice
- 1 tablespoon Dijon mustard
- 1 clove garlic, minced
- 1/2 teaspoon dried oregano
- Salt and pepper to taste

INSTRUCTIONS

1. Cook the Chicken: Preheat a grill or grill pan to medium-high heat. Rub chicken with 1 tablespoon olive oil, salt, and pepper. Grill for 5-7 minutes per side, or until cooked through. Let rest for 5 minutes before slicing thinly.

2. Make the Vinaigrette: In a small bowl or jar, whisk together olive oil, lemon juice, Dijon mustard, garlic, oregano, salt, and pepper.

3. Assemble the Salad: In a large bowl, combine spiralized zucchini, tomatoes, cucumber, sliced chicken, and feta (optional).

4. Dress & Serve: Pour vinaigrette over salad and toss to coat. Serve immediately or chill.

- No Spiralizer? Buy pre-spiralized zucchini noodles, or thinly slice the zucchini into ribbons.

- Make it Vegetarian: Swap grilled chicken for crispy tofu or chickpeas for a protein-rich vegetarian option.

- Add More Veggies: Feel free to include other vegetables like bell peppers, onions, or olives.

NUTRITIONAL FACTS

- Calories: 300

- Protein: 35 g

- Fat: 16 g

- Total Carbohydrates: 10 g

- Net Carbohydrates: 7 g

- Fiber: 3 g

ASIAN TURKEY LETTUCE WRAPS

Yields: 4 servings | **Prep Time:** 10 minutes | **Cook Time:** 15 minutes | **Total Time:** 25 minutes

INGREDIENTS

- 1 tablespoon olive oil
- 1 pound ground turkey
- 1/2 cup chopped onion
- 1 cup shredded carrots
- 1 (8-ounce) can water chestnuts, drained and chopped
- 1/4 cup hoisin sauce
- 2 tablespoons soy sauce (or use tamari or coconut aminos
- 1 tablespoon rice vinegar
- 1 teaspoon grated fresh ginger
- 1/2 teaspoon sesame oil
- 1/4 teaspoon red pepper flakes (optional)
- 12 large lettuce leaves (butter lettuce or iceberg work well)
- Toppings: sliced green onions, chopped peanuts, sriracha (optional)

INSTRUCTIONS

1. **Cook the Filling:** Heat olive oil in a large skillet over medium-high heat. Add ground turkey and onion, breaking up the meat with a spoon. Cook until the turkey is browned and the onion is softened, about 5-7 minutes.

2. **Add Veggies & Sauces:** Stir in shredded carrots, water chestnuts, hoisin sauce, soy sauce, rice vinegar, ginger, sesame oil, and red pepper flakes (if using). Cook for an additional 2-3 minutes, or until the sauce thickens slightly.

3. **Assemble the Wraps:** Spoon the turkey mixture into lettuce leaves. Top with desired toppings like sliced green onions, chopped peanuts, and sriracha. Serve immediately.

TIPS

TIPS

- Spice It Up: Adjust the red pepper flakes for desired heat.
- Vegetarian Option: Substitute crumbled extra-firm tofu for the ground turkey.
- Make it a Meal: Serve with a side of cauliflower rice or a small portion of brown rice for a heartier lunch.

NUTRITIONAL FACTS

Calories: 320

Protein: 26 g

Fat: 16 g

Total Carbohydrates: 22 g

Net Carbohydrates: 17 g

Fiber: 5 g

STEAK SALAD WITH BLUE CHEESE & BALSAMIC

Yields: 4 servings **Prep Time:** 10 minutes **Cook Time:** 10-15 minutes (depending on desired steak doneness) **Total Time:** 20-25 minutes

INGREDIENTS

- 1 pound flank steak (or your preferred cut)
- 1 tablespoon olive oil
- Salt and black pepper to taste
- 4 cups mixed greens or arugula
- 1/2 cup crumbled blue cheese
- 1/2 cup cherry tomatoes, halved
- 1/4 cup sliced red onion

Balsamic Vinaigrette:

- 3 tablespoons olive oil
- 2 tablespoons balsamic vinegar
- 1 teaspoon Dijon mustard
- 1/4 teaspoon honey (or other low-carb sweetener, optional)
- Salt and pepper to taste

INSTRUCTIONS

1. **Cook the Steak:** Season the steak generously with salt and pepper. Heat olive oil in a large skillet (preferably cast iron) over medium-high heat. Add the steak and cook to your desired doneness, about 3-5 minutes per side for medium-rare. Remove from pan and let rest for 5 minutes before thinly slicing against the grain.

2. **Make the Vinaigrette:** In a small bowl or jar, whisk together olive oil, balsamic vinegar, Dijon mustard, honey (if using), salt, and pepper.

3. **Assemble the Salad:** Divide the greens among 4 plates. Top with sliced steak, blue cheese, tomatoes, and red onion.

4. **Dress & Serve:** Drizzle the balsamic vinaigrette over the salads and serve immediately.

- Customize Your Steak: Use your favorite cut of steak, like sirloin, ribeye, or skirt steak.

- No Grill? No Problem! You can cook the steak in a skillet like the recipe outlines.

- Make it Ahead: Cook the steak and make the vinaigrette in advance for quick assembly during lunch breaks.

NUTRITIONAL FACTS

- Calories: 380

- Protein: 30 g

- Fat: 28 g

- Total Carbohydrates: 7 g

- Net Carbohydrates: 5 g

- Fiber: 2 g

LOW-CARB CHICKEN COBB SALAD

Yields: 4 servings **Prep Time:** 15 minutes **Cook Time:** 10-15 minutes (for chicken & eggs)

Total Time: 25-30 minutes

INGREDIENTS

- 1 pound boneless, skinless chicken breasts, grilled and sliced
- 4 cups mixed greens or romaine lettuce
- 4 hard-boiled eggs, sliced
- 1/2 cup crumbled bacon
- 1 avocado, sliced
- 1 cup cherry tomatoes, halved
- 1/2 cup crumbled blue cheese (or your preference)

Dressing Options:

- **Creamy Ranch:** Whisk together 1/2 cup mayonnaise, 1/4 cup sour cream (or Greek yogurt), 1 tablespoon white wine vinegar, 1/2 teaspoon dried dill, 1/4 teaspoon garlic powder, and salt and pepper to taste.
- **Blue Cheese Vinaigrette:** Whisk together 3 tablespoons olive oil, 2 tablespoons white wine vinegar, 2 tablespoons crumbled blue cheese, a pinch of Dijon mustard, and salt and pepper to taste.

INSTRUCTIONS

1. **Prep Your Ingredients:** Cook and slice your chicken, hard-boil and slice your eggs, and crumble your bacon.

2. **Assemble the Salad:** Divide the lettuce among 4 bowls or plates. Top with chicken, eggs, bacon, avocado, tomatoes, and cheese.

3. **Dress & Serve:** Drizzle with your preferred dressing and enjoy immediately!

- Make it Ahead: Prep the chicken, eggs, and dressing in advance. Assemble right before serving.
- Customize It: Add other low-carb veggies like cucumbers, bell peppers, or sliced radishes for extra crunch.

NUTRITIONAL FACTS (Without Dressings)

- Calories: 350
- Protein: 38 g
- Fat: 25 g
- Total Carbohydrates: 7 g
- Net Carbohydrates: 5 g
- Fiber: 2 g

TUNA SALAD WITH CUCUMBER "CRACKERS"

Yields: 2-3 servings | (depending on serving size) **Prep Time:** 10 minutes | **Total Time:** 10 minutes

INGREDIENTS

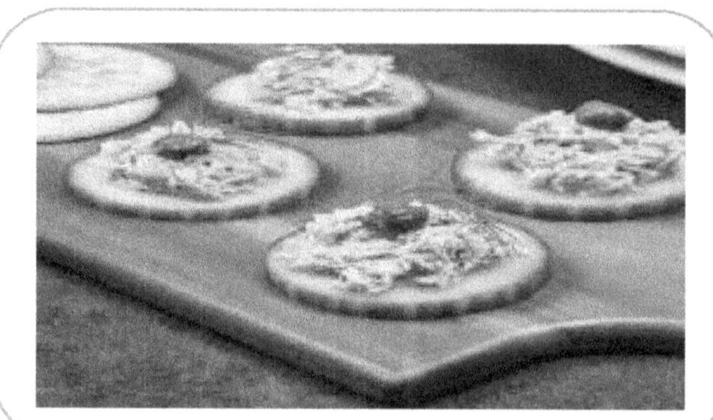

- 1 (5-ounce) can tuna, drained and flaked
- 1/4 cup mayonnaise (or plain Greek yogurt)
- 2 tablespoons chopped celery
- 1 tablespoon chopped fresh dill (or 1 teaspoon dried dill)
- 1 tablespoon lemon juice
- Salt and pepper to taste
- 1 medium cucumber, sliced into thick rounds

INSTRUCTIONS

1. **Make the Tuna Salad:** In a medium bowl, combine tuna, mayonnaise (or yogurt), celery, dill, lemon juice, salt, and pepper. Mix well.

2. **Assemble:** Serve immediately with cucumber slices as "crackers" for scooping up the tuna salad.

TIPS

- Get Creative with Add-Ins: Stir in chopped hard-boiled eggs, capers, olives, or finely diced red onion for variations.
- Storage: Tuna salad can be stored in an airtight container in the refrigerator for up to 3 days.

NUTRITIONAL FACTS (Approximate, Per Serving Without Cucumber Crackers)

- Calories: 200
- Protein: 22g
- Fat: 14 g
- Total Carbohydrates: 2 g
- Net Carbohydrates: 1g
- Fiber: 1g

ROAST BEEF AND HAVARTI ROLL-UPS

Yields: 4 servings | **Prep time:** 5 minutes | **Total Time:** 5 minutes

INGREDIENTS

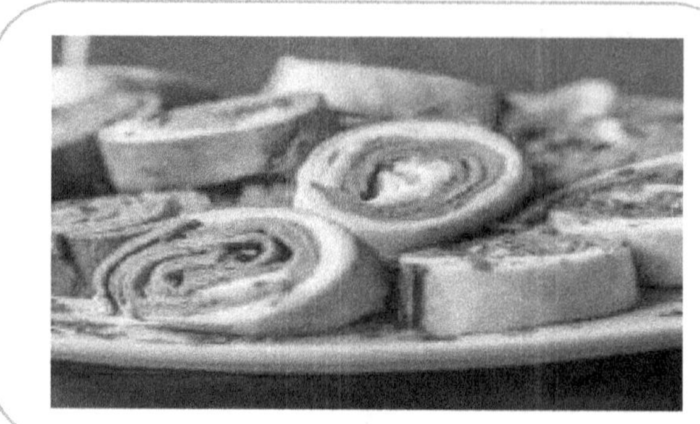

- 8 thin slices roast beef
- 4 slices Havarti cheese
- Optional: Dijon mustard, horseradish
- Lettuce leaves for freshness

INSTRUCTIONS

1. **Roll It Up:** Lay out roast beef slices and top each with a slice of Havarti. If using, add a thin smear of Dijon mustard or horseradish. Roll up tightly.
2. **Serve:** Place roll-ups on lettuce leaves for extra freshness and crunch. Enjoy immediately or store in the fridge for a grab-and-go lunch.

TIPS

- Customize It: Swap the roast beef for turkey pastrami, ham, or other thinly sliced deli meats.
- Veggie Boost: Add a few arugula leaves or a sprinkle of sprouts inside the roll-ups.

NUTRITIONAL FACTS

- Calories: 180
- Protein: 18 g
- Fat: 12 g
- Total Carbohydrates: 2 g
- Net Carbohydrates: 1 g
- Fiber: 1 g

Yields: 2 servings | **Prep Time:** 15 minutes | **Total Time:** 15 minutes (plus a few hours chilling time)

INGREDIENTS

- 2 (5-ounce) cans or pouches of salmon, drained
- 4 cups mixed greens or spinach
- 1 cup sliced cucumber
- 1/2 cup cherry tomatoes, halved
- 1/4 cup thinly sliced red onion
- Optional: 1/4 cup crumbled feta or goat chees

Vinaigrette:

- 3 tablespoons extra virgin olive oil
- 2 tablespoons lemon juice
- 1 teaspoon Dijon mustard
- 1/2 teaspoon dried oregano
- Salt and pepper to taste

INSTRUCTIONS

1. **Make the Vinaigrette:** In a small jar with a lid, whisk together olive oil, lemon juice, Dijon, oregano, salt, and pepper.

2. **Layer the Salad:** Divide the ingredients between two wide-mouth mason jars (pint size or larger). Layer in this order:

   o Dressing (about 2 tablespoons per jar)

   o Cucumber

   o Cherry tomatoes

   o Red onion

   o Salmon

   o Greens (lightly pressed to fit the jar)

   o Optional: cheese

3. **Chill & Serve:** Seal the jars tightly and refrigerate for at least a few hours, or up to 3 days. When ready to eat, shake the jar vigorously to distribute the dressing and then either eat directly from the jar or pour into a bowl.

TIPS

- Keep It Crisp: Layer ingredients in the order above to ensure the greens stay fresh and don't become soggy from the dressing prematurely.
- Protein Swap: Use grilled chicken or shrimp instead of salmon.
- Customize Your Veggie Combo: Add other low-carb favorites like sliced bell peppers, radishes, or olives.

NUTRITIONAL FACTS

- Calories: 340
- Protein: 28 g
- Fat: 26 g
- Total Carbohydrates: 7 g
- Net Carbohydrates: 5 g
- Fiber: 2 g

STEAK & ROASTED VEGGIE BOWL

Yields: 4 servings | **Prep Time:** 15 minutes | **Cook Time:** 20-25 minutes (depending on desired steak doneness) | **Total Time:** 35 - 40 minutes

INGREDIENTS

- 1 pound flank steak (or your preferred cut), thinly sliced
- 1 tablespoon olive oil
- Salt and pepper to taste
- 2 bell peppers (any color), sliced
- 1 medium onion, sliced
- 1 head broccoli, cut into florets
- 2 tablespoons olive oil
- 1 teaspoon garlic powder
- 1/2 teaspoon paprika

Optional Creamy Garlic-Herb Sauce:

- 1/2 cup plain Greek yogurt
- 1 tablespoon lemon juice
- 2 tablespoons chopped fresh herbs (parsley, dill, chives, or a mix)
- 1 clove garlic, minced
- Salt and pepper to taste

INSTRUCTIONS

1. **Season & Sear the Steak:** Season steak generously with salt and pepper. Heat 1 tablespoon of olive oil in a large skillet over medium-high heat. Add steak and sear until browned on both sides and cooked to your desired doneness. Let rest for 5 minutes before slicing thinly.

2. **Roast the Veggies:** Preheat oven to 425°F (220°C). Toss bell peppers, onion, and broccoli florets with olive oil, garlic powder, paprika, and salt and pepper. Roast on a baking sheet for 15-20 minutes, or until crisp-tender and slightly browned.

3. **Make the Sauce (Optional):** Whisk together Greek yogurt, lemon juice, herbs, garlic, salt, and pepper in a small bowl.

4. **Assemble the Bowls:** Divide the roasted vegetables among 4 bowls. Top with sliced steak. Drizzle with the creamy garlic-herb sauce (if using).

- *Customize Your Protein:* Swap the steak for grilled chicken, shrimp, or tofu.
- Experiment with Veggies: Add carrots, Brussels sprouts, asparagus – use your favorites!
- Make it Ahead: Prep and roast your veggies in advance. Sear the steak when ready to assemble.

NUTRITIONAL FACTS

- Calories: 320
- Protein: 30 g
- Fat: 18 g
- Total Carbohydrates: 12 g
- Net Carbohydrates: 7 g
- Fiber: 5 g

NICOISE SALAD

Yields: 4 servings | **Prep Time:** 15 minutes | **Cook Time:** 10-15 minutes | **Total Time:** 25 -30 minutes

INGREDIENTS

- 1 pound green beans, trimmed
- 4 large eggs
- 1 (5-ounce) can or pouch tuna, drained
- 1/2 cup cherry tomatoes, halved
- 1/4 cup sliced black olives
- 2 tablespoons capers (optional)
- 4 cups mixed greens
- Optional: 1/4 cup roasted cauliflower florets (for a subtle nod to potatoes)

Dijon Vinaigrette:

- 3 tablespoons extra virgin olive oil
- 2 tablespoons Dijon mustard
- 1 tablespoon lemon juice
- 1 clove garlic, minced
- Salt and pepper to taste

INSTRUCTIONS

1. **Cook Veggies & Eggs:** Bring a pot of salted water to a boil. Cook green beans for 3-5 minutes, or until crisp-tender. Drain and rinse with cold water. Boil eggs for 8-10 minutes, then transfer to ice water. Peel and cut into quarters.

2. **Make the Vinaigrette:** In a small jar, whisk together olive oil, Dijon, lemon juice, garlic, salt, and pepper.

3. **Assemble the Salad:** Divide mixed greens among 4 bowls. Top with green beans, quartered eggs, tuna, tomatoes, olives, capers (if using), and optional roasted cauliflower florets.

4. **Dress & Serve:** Drizzle vinaigrette over the salad and enjoy immediately.

- Grill It: For extra flavor, grill the green beans instead of boiling.

- Swap the Tuna: Use grilled salmon or chicken for a different twist.

- Make it Ahead: Cook the green beans, eggs, and roast the cauliflower in advance. Assemble right before serving.

NUTRITIONAL FACTS

- Calories: 300
- Protein: 25 g
- Fat: 22 g
- Total Carbohydrates: 9 g
- Net Carbohydrates: 6 g
- Fiber: 3 g

SPICY COCONUT CURRY WITH CHICKEN & CAULIFLOWER

Yields: 4 servings | **Prep Time:** 15 minutes | **Cook Time:** 25-30 minutes | **Total Time:** 40-45 minutes

INGREDIENTS

- 1 tablespoon olive oil
- 1 pound boneless, skinless chicken breasts, cut into bite-sized pieces
- 1 medium onion, chopped
- 1 head of cauliflower, cut into florets
- 2 bell peppers (any color), chopped
- 2 cloves garlic, minced
- 1 tablespoon grated fresh ginger
- 1-2 teaspoons curry powder (adjust for desired spice level)
- 1/2 teaspoon turmeric powder
- 1/4 teaspoon cayenne pepper (optional, for extra heat)
- 1 (14.5 ounce) can full-fat coconut milk
- 1 (14.5 ounce) can diced tomatoes, undrained
- 1/2 cup vegetable broth
- Salt and pepper to taste
- Chopped fresh cilantro for garnish (optional)

INSTRUCTIONS

1. **Sauté the Chicken and Aromatics:** Heat olive oil in a large pot over medium-high heat. Add chicken, season with salt and pepper, and cook until browned on all sides. Remove chicken and set aside. Add onion, garlic, and ginger to the pot and cook until softened, about 5 minutes.

2. **Add Spices and Cauliflower:** Stir in curry powder, turmeric, and cayenne (if using). Add cauliflower florets and bell peppers and cook for an additional 2-3 minutes, or until slightly softened.

3. **Simmer the Curry:** Return the chicken to the pot, along with coconut milk, diced tomatoes, and vegetable broth. Bring to a simmer, then reduce heat, cover, and cook for 15-20 minutes, or until chicken is cooked through and cauliflower is tender.

4. **Season & Serve:** Season with salt and pepper to taste. Serve hot, garnished with fresh cilantro (if desired), over cauliflower rice (if desired) or on its own.

TIPS

- Veg It Up: Add other low-carb veggies like broccoli, spinach, or zucchini.
- Make it Ahead: Curry flavors intensify over time – it's even better the next day!
- Customize the Spice: Adjust curry powder and cayenne to your heat preference.

NUTRITIONAL FACTS

- Calories: 380
- Protein: 35 g
- Fat: 24 g
- Total Carbohydrates: 14 g
- Net Carbohydrates: 9 g
- Fiber: 5 g

Yields: 4 servings | **Prep Time:** 15 minutes | **Cook Time:** 10-15 minutes (for chicken) | **Total Time:** 25-30 minutes

INGREDIENTS

- 1 pound boneless, skinless chicken breasts, grilled and sliced
- 4 cups mixed greens or romaine lettuce
- 4 hard-boiled eggs, sliced
- 1/2 cup crumbled bacon
- 1 avocado, sliced
- 1 cup cherry tomatoes, halved
- 1/2 cup crumbled blue cheese (or your preference)
- 1/4 cup chopped walnuts
- 1/4 cup chopped almonds
- 1/4 cup sunflower seeds

Dressing Options:

- Creamy Ranch: Whisk together 1/2 cup mayonnaise, 1/4 cup sour cream (or Greek yogurt), 1 tablespoon white wine vinegar, 1/2 teaspoon dried dill, 1/4 teaspoon garlic powder, and salt and pepper to taste.
- Blue Cheese Vinaigrette: Whisk together 3 tablespoons olive oil, 2 tablespoons white wine vinegar, 2 tablespoons crumbled blue cheese, a pinch of Dijon mustard, and salt and pepper to taste.

INSTRUCTIONS

1. **Prep Your Ingredients:** Cook and slice your chicken, hard-boil and slice your eggs, crumble your bacon, and chop your nuts and seeds.

2. **Assemble the Salad:** Divide the lettuce among 4 bowls or plates. Top with chicken, eggs, bacon, avocado, tomatoes, cheese, and the nut/seed mix.

3. **Dress & Serve:** Drizzle with your preferred dressing and enjoy immediately!

Yields: 4 servings | **Prep Time:** 15 minutes + marinating time | **Cook Time:** 10-15 minutes (for chicken) | **Total Time:** 25-30 minutes (plus marinating)

INGREDIENTS

- Chicken Marinade:
  - 1 pound boneless, skinless chicken breasts, sliced or cut into chunks
  - 1/4 cup olive oil
  - 2 tablespoons lemon juice
  - 1 tablespoon dried oregano
  - 1 teaspoon garlic powder
  - 1/2 teaspoon salt
  - 1/4 teaspoon black pepper
- Salad:
  - 1 cup sliced cucumber
  - 1 cup cherry tomatoes, halved
  - 1/2 cup sliced red onion
  - 1/2 cup crumbled feta cheese
  - 1/4 cup kalamata olives, sliced

- Dressing:
  - 3 tablespoons olive oil
  - 2 tablespoons red wine vinegar
  - 1 teaspoon Dijon mustard
  - 1 teaspoon dried oregano
  - 1/2 teaspoon garlic powder (optional)
  - Salt and pepper to taste

INSTRUCTIONS

1. **Marinate the Chicken:**

   - Combine olive oil, lemon juice, oregano, garlic powder, salt, and pepper in a bowl or ziplock bag.

o Add chicken and marinate for at least 30 minutes, or up to overnight for maximum flavor.

2. **Grill the Chicken:**

    o Preheat a grill or grill pan to medium-high heat.

    o Grill the marinated chicken until cooked through, about 5-7 minutes per side depending on thickness.

    o Let cool slightly and slice or chop.

3. **Make the Dressing:**

    o Whisk together the olive oil, red wine vinegar, Dijon mustard, oregano, garlic powder (if using), salt and pepper in a small bowl or jar.

4. **Assemble the Salad:**

    o In a large bowl, combine the grilled chicken, cucumber, tomatoes, red onion, feta cheese, and olives.

    o Pour the dressing over the salad and toss to coat.

5. **Serve:** Enjoy immediately or chill for later.

TIPS

- Extra Flavor: Add capers or a sprinkle of dried dill for more Mediterranean flair.
- Make It a Meal: Serve on top of greens, or with a small portion of roasted cauliflower florets for a heartier lunch.
- Grill It All: Grill or roast the vegetables too, along with the chicken, for an even greater depth of flavor.

NUTRITIONAL FACTS

- Calories: 310
- Protein: 35 g
- Fat: 20 g

- Total Carbohydrates: 6 g

- Net Carbohydrates: 4 g

- Fiber: 2 g

CHAPTER SEVEN

DINNER DELIGHTS

SHRIMP SCAMPI WITH ZUCCHINI NOODLES

Yields: 4 servings | **Prep Time:** 10 minutes | **Cook Time:** 10-12 minutes | **Total Time:** 20-22 minutes

INGREDIENTS

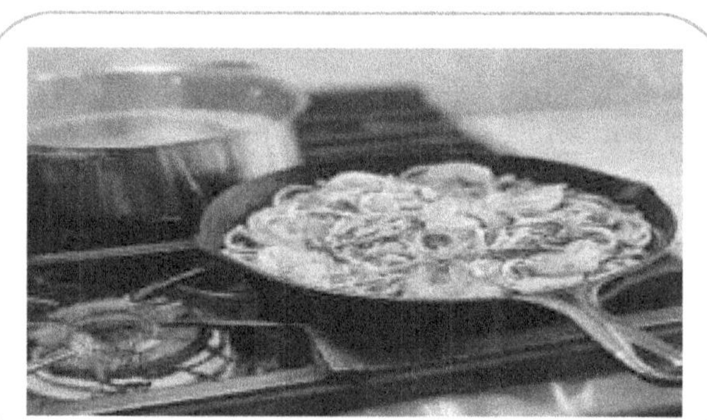

- 1 pound large shrimp, peeled and deveined
- 1 tablespoon olive oil
- 4 cloves garlic, minced
- 1/2 teaspoon red pepper flakes (optional, for heat)
- 1/4 cup dry white wine
- 1/4 cup lemon juice
- 3 tablespoons butter, cut into cubes
- 1/4 cup chopped fresh parsley
- 4 medium zucchini, spiralized
- Salt and pepper to taste

INSTRUCTIONS

1. Prep the Zoodles: Spiralize the zucchini. Pat the "noodles" dry with a paper towel to remove excess moisture.

2. Cook the Shrimp: Heat the olive oil in a large skillet over medium-high heat. Add the shrimp, season with salt and pepper, and cook for 2-3 minutes per side, or until pink and cooked through. Remove the shrimp and set aside.

3. Make the Sauce: Add the garlic and red pepper flakes (if using) to the skillet and cook for 30 seconds, or until fragrant. Deglaze the pan with the white wine and lemon juice, scraping up any browned bits. Bring to a simmer.

4. Finish & Serve: Reduce heat to low and whisk in the butter, one cube at a time, until melted and sauce is creamy. Stir in parsley. Add the shrimp and zucchini noodles, tossing to coat. Cook for 1-2 minutes, or just until zoodles are slightly softened. Season with salt and pepper, and serve immediately.

TIPS

- Don't Overcook: Shrimp cook quickly! Overcooked shrimp become tough.
- Zoodle Options: If you don't have a spiralizer, use a vegetable peeler to create long, wide ribbons.
- Make it Spicy: Add more red pepper flakes for extra heat.

NUTRITIONAL FACTS

- Calories: 280
- Protein: 26 g
- Fat: 18 g
- Total Carbohydrates: 9 g
- Net Carbohydrates: 6 g
- Fiber: 3 g

BAKED COD WITH LEMON & CAPERS

Yields: 4 servings | **Prep Time:** 5 minutes | **Cook Time:** 15-20 minutes (depending on cod thickness) | **Total Time:** 20-25 minutes

INGREDIENTS

- 4 (6-ounce) cod fillets
- 2 tablespoons olive oil
- 1 lemon, thinly sliced
- 2 tablespoons capers, rinsed
- 2 tablespoons butter, melted
- 1/4 cup chopped fresh parsley (optional)
- Salt and pepper to taste

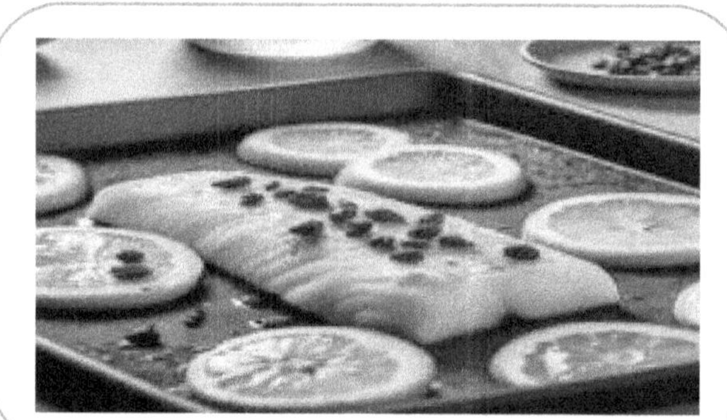

INSTRUCTIONS

1. **Preheat & Prep:** Preheat oven to 400°F (200°C). Lightly grease a baking dish. Arrange cod fillets in the dish.

2. **Top & Bake:** Drizzle olive oil over the cod. Top with lemon slices and capers. Pour over melted butter. Season with salt and pepper. Bake for 15-20 minutes, or until fish is opaque and flakes easily with a fork.

3. **Garnish & Serve:** Sprinkle with parsley (if using) and serve immediately.

- Parchment Paper: For easy cleanup, line the baking dish with parchment paper before adding the cod.
- Fresh Herbs: Substitute parsley with other fresh herbs like dill or thyme.
- Buttery Boost: Drizzle with extra melted butter just before serving for extra richness.

NUTRITIONAL FACTS

Calories: 250

Protein: 32 g

Fat: 15 g

Total Carbohydrates: 3 g

Net Carbohydrates: 2 g

Fiber: 1 g

SPICY SHRIMP TACOS WITH AVOCADO SALSA

Yields: 4 servings (about 3 tacos each) **Prep Time:** 15 minutes **Cook Time:** 10 minutes **Total Time:** 25 minutes

INGREDIENTS

- Shrimp:
  - 1 pound large shrimp, peeled and deveined
  - 1 tablespoon olive oil
  - 1 teaspoon chili powder
  - 1/2 teaspoon cumin
  - 1/4 teaspoon smoked paprika (optional)
  - 1/4 teaspoon garlic powder
  - Salt and pepper to taste
- Avocado Salsa:
  - 1 ripe avocado, diced
  - 1/2 cup cherry tomatoes, halved or quartered
  - 1/4 cup chopped red onion
  - 2 tablespoons chopped fresh cilantro
  - 2 tablespoons lime juice
  - 1/4 teaspoon salt
- Toppings:
  - Low-carb tortillas or lettuce leaves
  - Shredded cabbage (optional)
  - Hot sauce, for serving

INSTRUCTIONS

1. **Cook the Shrimp:** Heat olive oil in a large skillet over medium-high heat. Season shrimp with chili powder, cumin, smoked paprika (optional), garlic powder, salt, and pepper. Cook for 2-3 minutes per side, or until pink and cooked through. Remove and set aside

2. **Make the Salsa:** In a medium bowl, combine avocado, tomatoes, onion, cilantro, lime juice, and salt. Gently mix.

3. **Assemble the Tacos:** Warm your low-carb tortillas (if using). Fill with shrimp, avocado salsa, and a sprinkle of shredded cabbage (if desired). Drizzle with your favorite hot sauce.

- Adjust the Spice: Customize the heat level by increasing or decreasing the chili powder.

- Lettuce Wraps: Use large lettuce leaves (like butter or romaine) for a satisfying low-carb taco.

- Make-Ahead Salsa: The salsa can be made a few hours in advance for flavors to meld.

NUTRITIONAL FACTS

Calories: 250

Protein: 25 g

Fat: 16 g

Total Carbohydrates: 10 g

Net Carbohydrates: 7 g

Fiber: 3 g

TUNA BURGERS WITH WASABI MAYO

Yields: 4 servings **Prep Time:** 10 minutes **Cook Time:** 10-12 minutes **Total Time:** 20-22 minutes

INGREDIENTS

- Tuna:
    - 2 (5-ounce) cans of tuna packed in water, drained and flaked
    - 1/4 cup finely chopped red onion
    - 2 tablespoons chopped fresh parsley (or 1 tablespoon dried parsley)
    - 1 large egg, lightly beaten
    - 1/4 teaspoon salt
    - 1/4 teaspoon black pepper
- Wasabi Mayo:
    - 1/4 cup mayonnaise
    - 1-2 teaspoons wasabi paste (adjust to your desired heat level)
- Toppings & Serving:
    - 4 low-carb buns or lettuce leaves
    - Sliced tomato
    - Sliced avocado
    - Additional lettuce

INSTRUCTIONS

1. **Make Tuna Patties:** In a medium bowl, combine tuna, onion, parsley, egg, salt, and pepper. Mix well. Form into four equal patties.

2. **Cook Patties:** Heat a drizzle of olive oil in a large skillet or grill pan over medium-high heat. Cook tuna patties for 5-6 minutes per side, or until golden brown and cooked through.

3. **Make Wasabi Mayo:** While the patties cook, whisk together mayonnaise and wasabi paste in a small bowl.

4. **Assemble Burgers:** Spread wasabi mayo on buns (if using) or lettuce leaves. Top with tuna burgers, tomato, avocado, and additional lettuce (if desired). Serve immediately.

- Panko Alternative: For a gluten-free crunch, use crushed pork rinds instead of breadcrumbs (keep them low-carb or use as a higher-carb day option)
- Flavor Boost: Add a squeeze of lemon juice or a dash of soy sauce to the tuna mixture for extra flavor.
- Grill It: Tuna burgers are delicious grilled! Cook them over medium-high heat on a well-oiled grill.

NUTRITIONAL FACTS

Calories: 240

Protein: 30 g

Fat: 14 g

Total Carbohydrates: 3 g

Net Carbohydrates: 2 g

Fiber: 1 g

GRILLED LAMB SKEWERS WITH CUCUMBER-YOGURT SAUCE

Yields: 4 servings **Prep Time:** 15 minutes + marinating time **Cook Time:** 10-12 minutes **Total Time:** 25-30 minutes + marinating time

INGREDIENTS

- Marinade:
    - 1/2 cup plain yogurt
    - 1/4 cup olive oil
    - 2 tablespoons lemon juice
    - 2 cloves garlic, minced
    - 1 teaspoon dried oregano
    - 1/2 teaspoon dried mint
    - 1/2 teaspoon salt
    - 1/4 teaspoon black pepper
- Lamb & Skewers:
    - 1 pound boneless lamb leg or shoulder, cut into 1-inch cubes
    - 8-12 wooden skewers (soaked in water for 30 minutes if grilling)
- Cucumber-Yogurt Sauce:
    - 1 cup plain Greek yogurt
    - 1/2 cup chopped cucumber
    - 1 tablespoon chopped fresh mint (or 1 teaspoon dried mint)
    - 1 tablespoon lemon juice
    - Salt and pepper to taste

INSTRUCTIONS

1. **Marinate the Lamb:** In a bowl or ziplock bag, whisk together the marinade ingredients. Add the lamb cubes and toss to coat. Refrigerate for at least 30 minutes, or up to overnight for maximum flavor.

2. **Make the Sauce:** While the lamb marinates, combine all sauce ingredients in a bowl and season with salt and pepper. Refrigerate until serving.

3. **Thread the Skewers:** Remove the lamb from the marinade and thread the cubes onto the soaked skewers.

4. **Grill the Lamb:** Preheat a grill or grill pan to medium-high heat. Grill the skewers for 3-5 minutes per side, or until cooked to your desired doneness (medium-rare to medium is ideal).

5. **Serve:** Serve the lamb skewers immediately with the cucumber-yogurt sauce for dipping.

TIPS

- Other Veggies: Thread bell peppers, onions, or cherry tomatoes onto the skewers along with the lamb.
- Make it Spicy: Add a pinch of red pepper flakes to the marinade for a touch of heat.
- No Grill? No Problem: Cook the skewers in a skillet over medium-high heat with a drizzle of olive oil.

NUTRITIONAL FACTS

- Calories: 320
- Protein: 35 g
- Fat: 20 g
- Total Carbohydrates: 7 g
- Net Carbohydrates: 5 g
- Fiber: 2g

TURKEY MEATBALLS WITH MARINARA & ZOODLES

Yields: 4 servings **Prep Time:** 15 minutes **Cook Time:** 30-35 minutes **Total Time:** 45-50 minutes

INGREDIENTS

- Meatballs:
  - 1 pound ground turkey (93% lean or leaner)
  - 1/2 cup grated Parmesan cheese
  - 1/4 cup chopped fresh parsley (or 1 tablespoon dried parsley)
  - 1 large egg, lightly beaten
  - 1 teaspoon Italian seasoning
  - 1/2 teaspoon salt
  - 1/4 teaspoon black pepper
- Marinara Sauce:
  - 1 (28-ounce) can crushed tomatoes
  - 1/2 cup chopped onion
  - 2 cloves garlic, minced
  - 1 teaspoon dried basil
  - 1/2 teaspoon dried oregano
  - Salt and pepper to taste
- Zoodles:
  - 4 medium zucchini, spiralized

INSTRUCTIONS

1. **Make the Meatballs:** Preheat oven to 400°F (200°C). In a large bowl, combine ground turkey, Parmesan, parsley, egg, Italian seasoning, salt, and pepper. Form into 1-inch meatballs. Place them on a lightly greased baking sheet. Bake for 20-25 minutes, or until cooked through.

2. **Make the Marinara:** While meatballs bake, sauté onion in olive oil in a large saucepan until softened. Add garlic, cook for 30 seconds. Stir in crushed tomatoes, basil, oregano, salt, and pepper. Bring to a simmer and cook for 10-15 minutes, or until slightly thickened.

3. **Cook Zoodles:** Briefly sauté zoodles in a drizzle of olive oil over medium-high heat, just until tender-crisp (1-2 minutes). Season with salt and pepper.

4. **Serve:** Place a bed of zoodles on plates, top generously with marinara sauce and meatballs. Garnish with extra Parmesan if desired.

TIPS

- Avoid Dry Meatballs: Don't overmix the meatball mixture. Use a gentle touch when forming them to help keep them juicy.
- Flavor Up Your Zoodles: Add a pinch of red pepper flakes with the salt and pepper for a hint of spice.
- Make Ahead: The meatballs and sauce can be made a day in advance for even bolder flavors.

NUTRITIONAL FACTS

Calories: 400

Protein: 32 g

Fat: 16 g

Total Carbohydrates: 22 g

Net Carbohydrates: 17 g

Fiber: 5 g

Yields: 4 servings **Prep Time:** 10 minutes **Cook Time:** 15-20 minutes **Total Time:** 25-30 minutes

INGREDIENTS

- Salmon:
    - 4 (6-ounce) salmon fillets, skin-on or skinless
    - 1 tablespoon olive oil
    - Salt and pepper to taste
- Asparagus:
    - 1 pound asparagus, tough ends trimmed
    - 1 tablespoon olive oil
    - Salt and pepper to taste
- Dill Sauce:
    - 1/4 cup butter
    - 2 tablespoons lemon juice
    - 1 tablespoon chopped fresh dill (or 1 teaspoon dried dill)
    - 1/4 teaspoon salt
    - 1/8 teaspoon black pepper

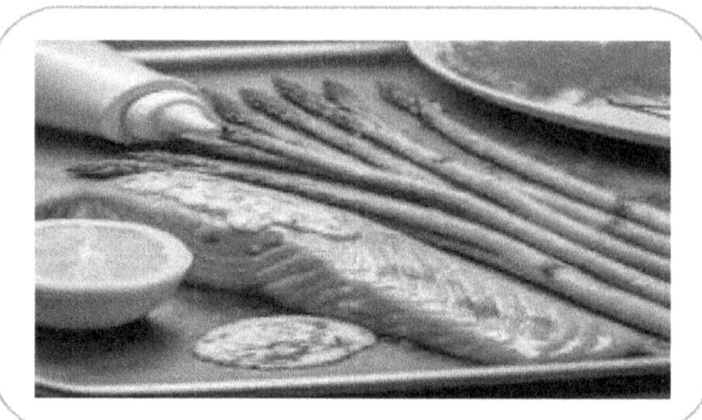

INSTRUCTIONS

1. Preheat Oven & Prep: Preheat oven to 425°F (220°C). Line a baking sheet with parchment paper. Arrange salmon fillets on one half of the sheet, drizzle with olive oil, and season with salt and pepper. Toss asparagus on the other half of the sheet with olive oil, salt, and pepper.

2. Roast Salmon & Asparagus: Roast for 12-15 minutes (depending on thickness), or until salmon is cooked through and flaky, and asparagus is tender-crisp.

3. Make the Sauce: While the salmon and asparagus cook, melt butter in a small saucepan over medium heat. Stir in lemon juice, dill, salt, and pepper.

4. Serve: Plate the roasted salmon and asparagus. Drizzle with the warm dill sauce and serve immediately.

TIPS

- Crispy Salmon Skin: For crispy skin, sear the salmon skin-side down in a skillet with olive oil for 2-3 minutes before transferring it to the baking sheet.
- Fresh Herb Substitutions: Use other fresh herbs like parsley, chives, or tarragon instead of dill.
- Lemony Boost: Add a touch of lemon zest to the sauce for a brighter flavor.

NUTRITIONAL FACTS

- Calories: 350
- Protein: 30 g
- Fat: 24 g
- Total Carbohydrates: 5 g
- Net Carbohydrates: 3 g
- Fiber: 2 g

CHICKEN STUFFED POBLANO PEPPERS

Yields: 4 servings **Prep Time:** 15 minutes **Cook Time:** 30-35 minutes **Total Time:** 45-50 minutes

INGREDIENTS

- Filling:
  - 1 tablespoon olive oil
  - 1/2 cup chopped onion
  - 1 pound ground chicken
  - 1 (4-ounce) can diced green chiles
  - 1 (10-ounce) can diced tomatoes & green chiles (like Rotel), undrained
  - 1/2 cup corn kernels (fresh or frozen)
  - 1/2 teaspoon cumin
  - 1/4 teaspoon chili powder
  - 1/4 teaspoon salt
  - 1/4 teaspoon black pepper
- Stuffed Peppers:
  - 4 medium poblano peppers, halved lengthwise, seeds and stems removed
  - 1 cup shredded Mexican cheese blend
- Optional Toppings:
  - Sour cream
  - Chopped fresh cilantro
  - Sliced avocado

INSTRUCTIONS

1. **Make the Filling:** Heat olive oil in a large skillet. Cook onion until softened. Add ground chicken, cook until browned. Drain excess grease. Stir in green chiles, tomatoes & chiles, corn, cumin, chili powder, salt, and pepper. Simmer for 5-10 minutes to combine flavors.

2. **Prep the Peppers:** Preheat oven to 400°F (200°C). Lightly grease a baking dish. Place pepper halves cut-side up in the prepared dish.

3. **Stuff & Bake:** Spoon chicken mixture into peppers. Top generously with cheese. Bake for 20-25 minutes, or until peppers are tender and cheese is melted and bubbly.

4. **Serve:** Let cool slightly. Top with sour cream, cilantro, and avocado (if desired).

- Spice It Up: Add a pinch of cayenne or your favorite hot sauce to the filling for extra heat.

- Dairy-Free: Use dairy-free cheese shreds or omit it entirely.

- Make Ahead: Prep the filling and stuff the peppers in advance. Refrigerate, then bake when ready.

- Calories: 300

- Protein: 30 g

- Fat: 15 g

- Total Carbohydrates: 17 g

- Net Carbohydrates: 13 g

- Fiber: 4 g

CREAMY MUSHROOM & SPINACH STUFFED CHICKEN

Yields: 4 servings **Prep Time:** 15 minutes **Cook Time:** 25-30 minutes **Total Time:** 40-45 minutes

INGREDIENTS

- 2 ripe avocados, pitted and diced
- 3 medium tomatillos, husked, rinsed, and diced
- ½ jalapeño pepper, seeded and finely chopped (adjust for desired spice level)
- ¼ cup finely chopped red onion
- 1 tablespoon fresh cilantro, chopped
- 1 tablespoon fresh lime juice
- ½ teaspoon sea salt
- Pinch of black pepper

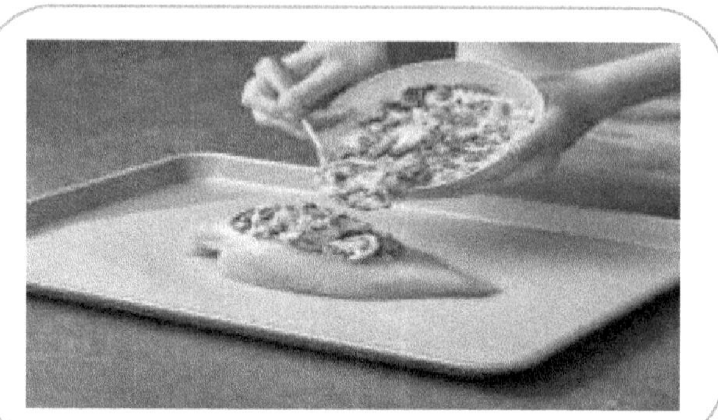

INSTRUCTIONS

1. **Prep the Chicken:** Preheat oven to 400°F (200°C). Butterfly each chicken breast by slicing it horizontally almost all the way through, then opening it like a book. Season with salt and pepper.

2. **Make the Filling:** Sauté mushrooms and onions in olive oil until softened. Stir in spinach, cream cheese, Parmesan, garlic powder, salt, and pepper, until well combined.

3. **Stuff & Bake:** Spread filling evenly among chicken breasts. Roll chicken up tightly and secure with toothpicks if needed. Bake for 25-30 minutes or until chicken is cooked through.

4. **Rest & Serve:** Let chicken rest for 5 minutes before slicing. Serve warm.

- Get Creative with Fillings: Add other mix-ins like artichoke hearts, roasted red peppers, or sundried tomatoes.
- Browning for Flavor: For an extra layer of flavor, sear the stuffed chicken breasts for a minute or two per side in a hot skillet before baking.
- Cheese Swap: Use your favorite melty cheese instead of Parmesan.

NUTRITIONAL FACTS

- Calories: 380
- Protein: 40 g
- Fat: 22 g
- Total Carbohydrates: 8 g
- Net Carbohydrates: 6 g
- Fiber: 2 g

ONE-PAN SAUSAGE & VEGGIE SKILLET

Yields: 4 servings **Prep Time:** 10 minutes **Cook Time:** 20-25 minutes **Total Time:** 30-35 minutes

INGREDIENTS

- 1 tablespoon olive oil
- 1 pound Italian sausage (sweet or spicy), casings removed (or use pre-cooked sausage)
- 1 medium onion, chopped
- 1 green bell pepper, chopped
- 1 red bell pepper, chopped
- 1 (14.5 ounce) can diced tomatoes, undrained
- 1 teaspoon Italian seasoning
- 1/2 teaspoon garlic powder
- 1/2 teaspoon salt
- 1/4 teaspoon black pepper

Optional but Delicious:

- 1/2 cup sliced mushrooms
- 1/2 cup zucchini, diced
- Freshly grated Parmesan cheese for serving

INSTRUCTIONS

1. **Brown the Sausage:** Heat olive oil in a large skillet over medium-high heat. Add sausage and cook, breaking it up with a spoon, until browned.

2. **Add the Veggies:** Add onion, bell peppers, and optional mushrooms or zucchini (if using). Cook for 5-7 minutes, or until vegetables soften.

3. **Season & Simmer:** Stir in diced tomatoes, Italian seasoning, garlic powder, salt, and pepper. Reduce heat to low and simmer for 10-15 minutes, or until sauce thickens slightly.

4. **Serve:** Taste and adjust seasonings. Serve hot, sprinkled with Parmesan cheese (if desired).

- Prep Ahead: Chop your vegetables in advance to make this even quicker.

- Make it Spicy: Use hot Italian sausage or add a pinch of red pepper flakes for a kick.

- Double Up: Easily double the recipe for leftovers or a larger crowd.

NUTRITIONAL FACTS

- Calories: 350

- Protein: 22 g

- Fat: 25 g

- Total Carbohydrates: 12 g

- Net Carbohydrates: 8 g

- Fiber: 4 g

AIR FRYER PORK CHOPS WITH PARMESAN CRUST

Yields: 4 servings | **Prep Time:** 5 minutes | **Cook Time:** 12-15 minutes | **Total Time:** 17-20 minutes

INGREDIENTS

- 4 boneless pork chops (about 1/2 inch thick)
- 1/4 cup grated Parmesan cheese
- 1 tablespoon Italian seasoning
- 1/2 teaspoon garlic powder
- 1/4 teaspoon salt
- 1/4 teaspoon black pepper

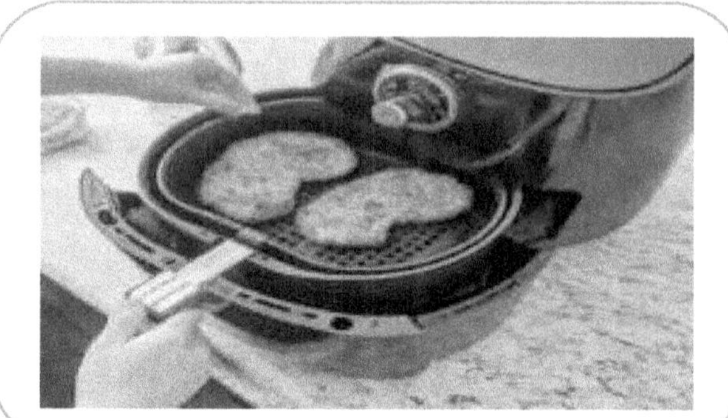

INSTRUCTIONS

1. **Preheat Air Fryer:** Preheat your air fryer to 400°F (200°C).

2. **Season Pork Chops:** Pat dry pork chops. In a shallow dish, combine Parmesan cheese, Italian seasoning, garlic powder, salt, and pepper. Coat both sides of the pork chops with the Parmesan mixture.

3. **Air Fry:** Place pork chops in a single layer in the air fryer basket. Cook for 12-15 minutes, or until cooked through and the crust is golden brown. (Internal temperature should reach 145°F)

4. **Serve:** Let pork chops rest for a few minutes. Serve immediately with your favorite low-carb sides.

TIPS

- Thicker Chops: For pork chops thicker than 1/2 inch, increase cooking time by a few minutes or until fully cooked.
- Flavor Boost: Add a pinch of red pepper flakes for a touch of heat.
- Side Suggestions: Serve with roasted broccoli, cauliflower rice, or a simple salad.

NUTRITIONAL FACTS

- Calories: 260
- Protein: 35 g
- Fat: 14 g
- Total Carbohydrates: 2 g
- Net Carbohydrates: 1 g
- Fiber: 1 g

STEAK FAJITA BOWLS

Yields: 4 servings | **Prep Time:** 10-15 minutes | **Cook Time:** 15-20 minutes | **Total Time:** 25-35 minutes

INGREDIENTS

- The Steak:
    - 1 pound flank steak or skirt steak
    - 1 tablespoon olive oil
    - 1 teaspoon fajita seasoning (store-bought or homemade)
    - Salt and pepper to taste
- The Veggies:
    - 1 tablespoon olive oil
    - 1 large onion, sliced
    - 1 green bell pepper, sliced
    - 1 red bell pepper, sliced
- For Serving:
    - Cauliflower rice (warmed)
    - Guacamole
    - Sour cream
    - Salsa
    - Chopped fresh cilantro

INSTRUCTIONS

1. **Prep & Marinate:** Pat dry steak and season with fajita seasoning, salt, and pepper. Let marinate for at least 15 minutes or up to overnight for bolder flavor.

2. **Cook the Veggies:** Heat olive oil in a large skillet over medium-high heat. Add onion and peppers, cook until softened, about 5-7 minutes. Season with salt and pepper. Remove from the skillet and set aside.

3. **Cook the Steak:** Heat the same skillet over high heat. Add steak and cook 3-5 minutes per side for medium-rare, adjust for desired doneness. Let rest for 5 minutes, then slice thinly against the grain.

4. **Assemble the Bowls:** Divide cauliflower rice between bowls. Top with steak, sauteed peppers and onions, guacamole, sour cream, salsa, and a sprinkle of cilantro.

TIPS

- Customize It: Add your favorite fajita toppings like shredded cheese, sliced avocado, or hot sauce.
- Alternate Protein: Swap steak for grilled chicken or shrimp.
- Make it Ahead: Cook steak and veggies a day in advance for quick assembly.

NUTRITIONAL FACTS

- Calories: 320
- Protein: 30 g
- Fat: 20g
- Total Carbohydrates: 10 g
- Net Carbohydrates: 7 g
- Fiber: 3 g

Yields: 4 servings **Prep Time:** 10 minutes **Cook Time:** 15-20 minutes **Total Time:** 25-30 minutes

INGREDIENTS

- Tofu:
  - 1 (14-ounce) block extra-firm tofu, drained and pressed
  - 1 tablespoon olive oil
  - 1/2 teaspoon chili powder
  - 1/4 teaspoon cumin
  - 1/4 teaspoon turmeric
  - 1/4 teaspoon salt
  - 1/8 teaspoon black pepper
- The Scramble:
  - 1/2 cup chopped onion
  - 1/2 cup chopped green bell pepper
  - 1 (15-ounce) can black beans, rinsed and drained
  - 1 cup salsa (choose your favorite mild, medium, or spicy)
- Toppings (Optional):
  - Chopped fresh cilantro
  - Sliced avocado
  - Hot sauce

INSTRUCTIONS

1. **Prep the Tofu:** Crumble the tofu into a bowl using your hands or a fork.

2. **Season the Tofu:** In a large skillet, heat olive oil over medium heat. Add crumbled tofu, chili powder, cumin, turmeric, salt, and pepper. Cook for 5-7 minutes, or until tofu is heated through and slightly browned, stirring occasionally.

3. **Add the Veggies & Beans:** Add onion and green bell pepper to the skillet. Cook for 3-5 minutes, or until softened. Stir in black beans and heat through.

4. **Finish & Serve:** Stir in salsa. Season to taste with additional salt and pepper. Serve hot, garnished with cilantro, avocado, and hot sauce (if desired).

- Press the Tofu: Pressing the tofu removes excess moisture and helps it achieve a better texture. Wrap the block in paper towels and place a heavy object on top for at least 30 minutes.
- Flavor Variations: Add other spices like garlic powder, smoked paprika, or a pinch of red pepper flakes for a kick.
- Make it Breakfast: Top a serving with a fried egg for a satisfying breakfast scramble.

NUTRITIONAL FACTS

- Calories: 250
- Protein: 15 g
- Fat: 12 g
- Total Carbohydrates: 22 g
- Net Carbohydrates: 14 g
- Fiber: 8 g

CHAPTER EIGHT

SNACKS & SWEET FIXES

ROASTED ALMONDS WITH HERBS & SPICES

Yields: 4 servings | **Prep Time:** 5 minutes | **Cook Time:** 10-15 minutes | **Total Time:** 15-20 minutes

INGREDIENTS

- 1 cup raw almonds
- 1 tablespoon olive oil
- 1 teaspoon of your favorite spice blend (ideas below)
- 1/2 teaspoon salt

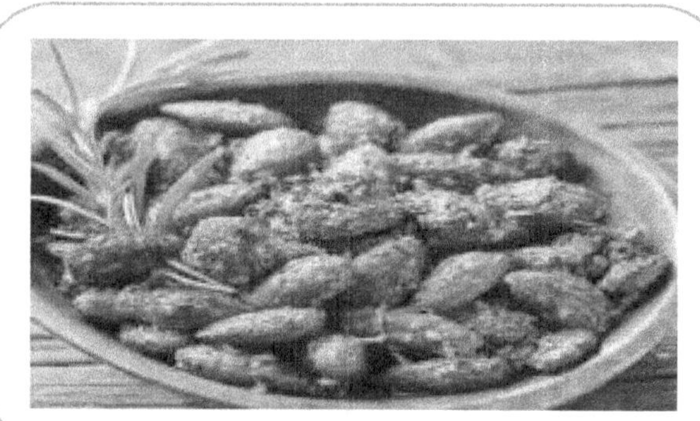

Spice Blend Options:

- Rosemary & Garlic: Dried rosemary, garlic powder, a pinch of black pepper
- Smoky Cajun: Smoked paprika, cayenne pepper, garlic powder, onion powder
- Sweet & Spicy: Cinnamon, chili powder, a tiny bit of your preferred low-carb sweetener.
- Simple & Savory: Just salt and pepper

INSTRUCTIONS

1. **Preheat & Prep:** Preheat oven to 350°F (175°C). Line a baking sheet with parchment paper.
2. **Season:** In a bowl, toss almonds with olive oil, your chosen spice blend, and salt. Spread them in a single layer on the prepared baking sheet.

3. **Roast & Enjoy:** Roast for 10-15 minutes, or until golden brown and fragrant. Stir halfway through cooking for even roasting. Let cool slightly before enjoying.

TIPS

- Experiment: Don't be afraid to experiment with different spice combinations. Get creative!
- Bulk It Up: Double or triple the recipe for a larger batch.
- Storage: Store cooled almonds in an airtight container at room temperature for up to 5 days.

NUTRITIONAL FACTS

Calories: 200

Protein: 6 g

Fat: 18 g

Total Carbohydrates: 6 g

Net Carbohydrates: 3 g

Fiber: 3 g

DEVILED EGGS WITH BACON CRUMBLES

Yield: 12 deviled egg halves | **Prep Time**: Approximately 15-20 minutes | **Cook Time**: 10-12 minutes (hard-boiling the eggs) | **Total Time**: Around 25-32 minutes

INGREDIENTS

- 6 large eggs
- 1/4 cup mayonnaise (use a full-fat variety for the most richness)
- 1 tablespoon Dijon mustard
- 1 teaspoon white vinegar or lemon juice
- 1/4 teaspoon salt
- 1/8 teaspoon black pepper
- 2-3 slices bacon, cooked and crumbled
- Optional: Paprika or chives for garnish

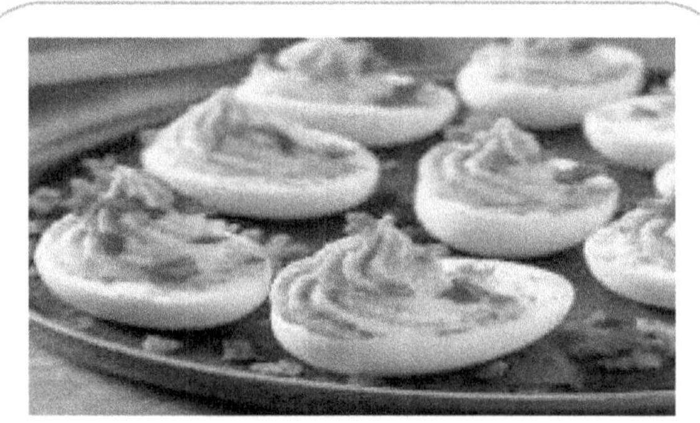

INSTRUCTIONS

1. **Hard Boil Eggs:** Place eggs in a pot and cover with cold water. Bring to a boil, cover, and remove from heat. Let sit for 10-12 minutes. Drain and cool in ice water. Peel shells carefully.

2. **Make Filling:** Slice eggs in half lengthwise. Scoop yolks into a bowl and mash with a fork. Add mayonnaise, mustard, vinegar (or lemon juice), salt, and pepper. Mix until smooth and creamy.

3. **Fill & Garnish:** Spoon or pipe filling back into egg white halves. Sprinkle with crumbled bacon and a dusting of paprika or chives (optional)

- Perfectly Cooked Eggs: For easy-to-peel eggs, use slightly older eggs. The air pocket gets larger, making them easier to peel.
- Creamy Filling: For an extra creamy filling, add a tablespoon of softened cream cheese to the yolk mixture.
- Flavor Boost: Try a little hot sauce or a pinch of smoked paprika in the yolk mixture.
- Make Ahead: Prep the filling and hard-boiled eggs a day ahead. Assemble just before serving.

NUTRITIONAL FACTS

Calories: 80

Protein: 5 g

Fat: 7 g

Total Carbohydrates: 1 g

Net Carbohydrates: 0.5 g

Fiber: 0.5 g

SAVORY YOGURT PARFAIT

Yields: 1 serving **Prep Time:** 5 minutes **Total Time:** 5 minutes

INGREDIENTS

* Base: 1/2 cup plain, full-fat Greek yogurt
* Toppings (Choose 2-3):
    * 1 tablespoon chopped fresh herbs (chives, dill, parsley, etc.)
    * 1 tablespoon crumbled cooked bacon
    * 1 tablespoon chopped nuts (almonds, walnuts, pecans)
    * 1 tablespoon chopped olives (Kalamata, green, etc.)
    * 1/2 teaspoon Everything Bagel seasoning
    * Pinch of red pepper flakes for heat (optional)

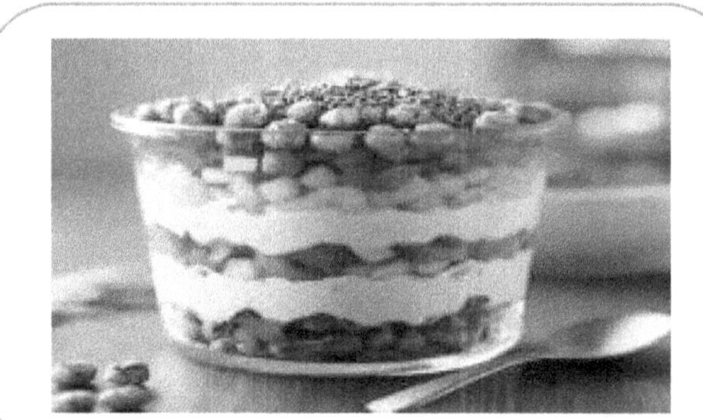

INSTRUCTIONS

1. Layer: In a small bowl or glass, layer the Greek yogurt with your chosen toppings.
2. Enjoy: Dig in immediately!

- Get Creative: Play around with different topping combinations to find your favorites.
- Make Ahead (Mostly): You can prep the toppings in advance and store them separately for quick assembly when you're ready to snack.
- Portion Control: This recipe is for one serving. To stay within your carb limits, stick to this portion size, or split it into two smaller snacks.

NUTRITIONAL FACTS

Calories: 150-200

Protein: 15-20g

Fat: 10-15g

Total Carbohydrates: 5-8g

Net Carbohydrates: 3-6g

Fiber: 2-3g

EVERYTHING" SPICED NUTS

Yields: 2 servings **Prep Time:** 5 minutes **Cook Time:** 10-12 minutes **Total Time:** 15-17 minutes

INGREDIENTS

- Nuts: 1/2 cup raw almonds, cashews, walnuts, or a mix
- Spice Mix:
    - 1 teaspoon dried minced onion
    - 1/2 teaspoon garlic powder
    - 1/2 teaspoon poppy seeds
    - 1/2 teaspoon sesame seeds
    - 1/4 teaspoon salt (or a generous pinch)
    - 1/8 teaspoon black pepper
- Optional:
    - Tiny drizzle of olive oil (helps spices stick, adds richness)
    - Pinch of cayenne pepper for a little heat

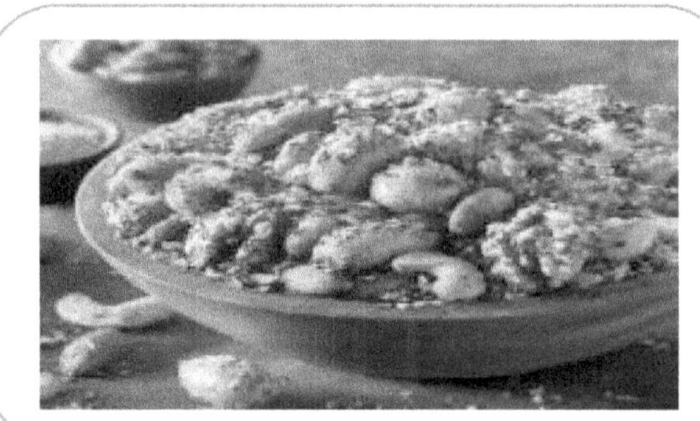

INSTRUCTIONS

1. **Preheat Oven:** Preheat oven to 350°F (175°C). Line a small baking sheet with parchment paper.

2. **Combine:** In a bowl, toss the nuts with the spice mix (and olive oil, if using).

3. **Roast:** Spread nuts in a single layer on the baking sheet. Roast for 10-12 minutes or until fragrant and lightly golden. Stir them halfway through for even roasting.

4. **Cool & Enjoy:** Let the nuts cool completely on the baking sheet before enjoying.

- Customize the Spices: This is a base recipe – get creative! Experiment with your favorite spice combinations.
- Bulk It Up: Double or triple the recipe for a larger batch.
- Storage: Store cooled nuts in an airtight container at room temperature for up to a week.

NUTRITIONAL FACTS

Calories: 200-250 (depending on nut type)

Protein: 8-10g

Fat: 18-22g

Total Carbohydrates: 6-8g

Net Carbohydrates: 3-5g

Fiber: 3-4g

TUNA OR SALMON SALAD "BOATS"

Yields: 2 servings **Prep Time:** 10 minutes **Total Time:** 10 minutes

INGREDIENTS

- Base: 4-5 small celery stalks, washed and trimmed
- Filling:
  - 5-ounce can of tuna or salmon, drained well
  - 1-2 tablespoons full-fat mayonnaise
  - 1 teaspoon Dijon mustard
  - 1/2 teaspoon lemon juice
  - 1/4 teaspoon salt
  - 1/8 teaspoon black pepper
- Optional Add-ins (choose 1-2):
  - 1 tablespoon finely chopped celery
  - 1 tablespoon finely chopped red onion
  - 1 teaspoon chopped fresh dill or parsley

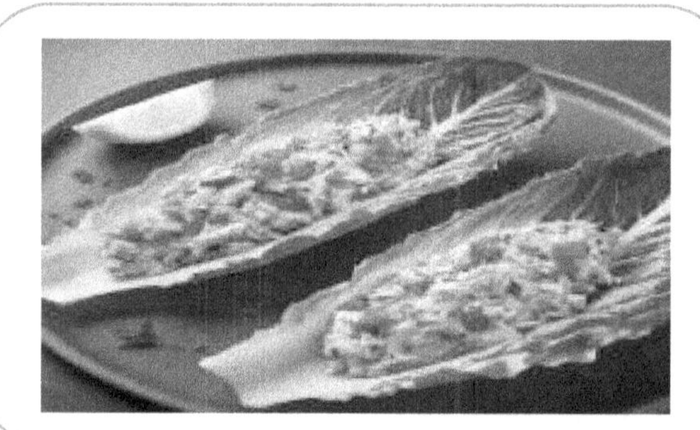

INSTRUCTIONS

1. **Make the Filling:** In a bowl, flake the tuna or salmon with a fork. Add mayonnaise, mustard, lemon juice, salt, and pepper. Mix well. Stir in any optional add-ins you like.

2. **Fill the "Boats":** Cut the celery stalks in half if desired. Fill each with a generous portion of the tuna or salmon salad.

3. **Enjoy!** Serve immediately for the best texture.

- Flavor Variations: Add a dash of hot sauce, a sprinkle of curry powder, or other spices you enjoy.
- Make it Crunchy: For extra texture, add chopped almonds or walnuts to the filling.
- Leftovers: Store leftover salad in an airtight container in the refrigerator for up to 2 days.

NUTRITIONAL FACTS

- Calories: 180-220
- Protein: 20-25g
- Fat: 12-16g
- Total Carbohydrates: 3-5g
- Net Carbohydrates: 1-3g
- Fiber: 2-3g

CHAPTER NINE

THE 21-DAY METABOLISM MAKEOVER

Understanding Your Calorie & Macro Needs

This plan isn't about severe restriction – it's about smart fueling. Let's demystify some numbers to empower your journey:

Basal Metabolic Rate (BMR)

Your body's resting metabolic expenditure to sustain essential bodily processes. It serves as your basic energy need. Your body needs energy for basic functions like breathing, circulation, nutrition processing, and cell production even while you're at rest. This is referred to as BMR, or basal metabolic rate.

Resting metabolic rate (RMR) and basal metabolic rate (BMR) are frequently used interchangeably. RMR, also known as resting energy expenditure (REE), is the amount of calories your body really burns while it is at rest, whereas BMR is the minimal amount of calories needed for fundamental processes at rest. Your RMR should be a reliable indicator of your BMR even though BMR and RMR differ slightly. The difference between the two figures is typically 10%.

How to estimate your BMR

The Harris-Benedict formula is a widely used method for estimating body mass index (BMR) and accounts for weight, height, age, and sex.

Females assigned at birth (FAABs)

BMR = 655 + (9.6 x weight in kg) + (1.8 x height in cm) – (4.7 x age in years)

Males assigned at birth (MAABs)

66 + (13.7 x weight in kg) + (5 x height in cm) – (6.8 x age in years)

Reasons to consider finding out your BMR

You can use your BMR to increase, decrease, or stay at your current weight. You can determine how many calories to eat by measuring how much you burn. To put it in easy terms:

- Do you want to keep your weight the same? Make sure you eat the same amount of calories as you expend.
- Do you want to put on weight? Eat more energy than you expend.
- Is weight loss your main objective? Eat less calories than you expend.

Other actors that can influence your weight. They include:

- your level of physical activity
- your sex
- your age
- any ailments you may have or drugs you currently take
- your metabolism
- your gut microbiome

Total Daily Energy Expenditure (TDEE)

This takes into consideration both your BMR and your amount of activity. We'll try to consume a little less than your TDEE in order to generate the calorie deficit required for fat loss. Thermic effect of food, exercise energy expenditure, basal metabolic rate, and non-exercise activity thermogenesis are the four numbers added together to determine total daily energy expenditure (TDEE).

TDEE = BMR + TEF + EEE + NEAT

Basal Metabolic Rate (BMR)
The amount of calories the body requires at rest for its organs to operate and to stay alive is known as the basal metabolic rate. The most precise method for calculating BMR is to use a device similar to an InBody. If you don't have access to one, you can calculate the person's weight in kilos by multiplying their body weight by 20.

Example:

176 pounds = 80 kg

80 kg x 20 = 1600

BMR of a 176 pound client = 1600 calories.

Thermic Effect of Feeding (TEF)

The amount of energy needed to digest the meal consumed must be factored in when calculating TDEE. Thermic effect of feeding is this. Just multiply the BMR by 0.1 to get TEF.

Example:

BMR = 1600

160 calories are burnt as a result of feeding (1600 x 0.1).

Exercise Energy Expenditure (EEE)

In the TDEE computation, exercise energy expenditure (EEE) is the third variable. This is how much energy is used up during exercising. Since everyone's EEE is different, it is impossible to calculate exactly, but as a general rule, it can range from 250 calories for moderate exercise to 500 for vigorous exercise.

Example:

An hour of exercise for a novice client equals 250 EEE.

500 EEE for an advanced customer exercising for at least an hour

Non-Exercise Activity Thermogenesis (NEAT)

The last and fourth variable is the thermogenesis of non-exercise activity (NEAT). This takes into consideration the amount of calories a client burns throughout their daily activities that do not involve physical activity, such as walking their dog, working manual labor, or spending all day at a desk job. Again, there is no precise figure for NEAT; it varies from 250 to 500 calories based on the amount of activity done during the day.

Example:

A sedentary desk job employee = 250 NEAT

A delivery driver or construction worker = 500 NEAT

Sample TDEE Calculation:

The client weighs 80 kg

BMR = 1600

TEF = 160

EEE = 250

NEAT = 250

TDEE 1600 + 160 + 250 + 250 = 2,260

Macronutrients – Your Body's Building Blocks

There are roles for lipids, carbs, and protein. We'll focus on a macro ratio designed for endomorph success: 40% protein, 30% carbohydrates, and 30% fats, for best outcomes on this diet. It's not important to hit this flawlessly every day; consistency over time is what matters most.

Endomorphs frequently gain from a higher protein diet in order to promote muscular growth and increase metabolism. By consciously limiting your intake of carbohydrates, you can help your body burn fat for energy and lose weight.

How to Calculate Macros Using TDEE

Since no two calories are the identical, one can divide calories into distinct macros after TDEE has been determined. The three primary nutrients that make up food are called macronutrients, or simply macros. These consist of lipids, carbs, and proteins. Knowing the precise macronutrient needs of individuals who have certain goals in mind—be they performance- or appearance-related—is beneficial. We will be working with a ratio of about 40% fat, 30% protein, and 40%

carbs in the example below. Although everyone has a different preferred ratio, it's worthwhile to experiment with several values to determine which one works best. This is a nice neutral starting point. There are a certain number of calories linked to each macronutrient: 4 calories are found in 1 gram of protein, 4 calories in 1 gram of carbs, and 9 calories in 1 gram of fat.

How to Calculate Protein Macros

Obtaining body weight or the weight of lean mass (if available) and activity levels is the first step in calculating protein macros. Usually, OPEX Coaches carry out this task during the evaluation. To determine their protein need, double their weight in lean mass by one to 1.5, depending on their degree of activity. In the event that you lack lean body mass, protein can be computed using weight. Take a first glance at your body fat percentage. Give yourself one gram of protein for every pound of body weight if your body fat percentage is 15% or less. To calculate their protein need, multiply bodyweight by.8 if their body fat percentage is more than 15%.

Example:

A customer weighing eighty-five pounds (175 kg)

Body fat = 12%

TDEE = 2260

175 pounds x 1 gram per pound of bodyweight = 175 grams of protein

At 4 calories per gram, 175 grams of protein is 700 calories, or just over 30% of TDEE.

How to Calculate Carbohydrate Macros

Since we are utilizing a 40/30/30 ratio in this example, we can determine our daily carbohydrate intake by dividing our TDEE by 40%. That would be 40% of 2260 in this instance. This works out to 904 calories. Consequently, 904 calories must come from carbs every day. After dividing that by 4, the daily amount of carbohydrates is 226 grams.

We will utilize the 40/30/30 split to compute fat macros once more. Since 30% of calories will be fat, we calculate that 30% of 2260 calories, or 678 calories, will be fat. Since there are 9 calories in every gram of fat, we now divide 678 calories by 9 to obtain 75 grams of fat.

Daily Macronutrient Goal for a 175 Pound Client:

Protein: 175 grams

Carbohydrate: 226 grams

Fat: 75 grams

WEEK 1

Day	Breakfast	Lunch	Dinner	Notes
Day 1	Cloud Eggs with Spinach & Feta (pg 23)	Steak Salad with Blue Cheese & Balsamic (pg 51)	Chicken Stuffed Poblano Peppers (pg 85)	
Day 2	Keto Frittata with Sausage & Peppers (pg 25)	Low-Carb Chicken Cobb Salad (pg 53)	Shrimp Scampi with Zucchini Noodles (pg 71)	
Day 3	Baked Eggs in Avocado with Smoked Salmon (pg 29)	Tuna Salad with Cucumber "Crackers" (pg 55)	Asian Turkey Lettuce Wraps (pg 49)	
Day 4	Crustless Broccoli & Cheddar Quiche (pg 27)	Mason Jar Salad with Salmon & Lemon Vinaigrette (pg 58)	Steak Fajita Bowls (pg 93)	Consider a slightly higher carb intake today.
Day 5	Shakshuka-Inspired Scramble with Chorizo (pg 31)	Roast Beef and Havarti Roll-Ups (pg 57)	Tuna Burgers with Wasabi Mayo (pg 77)	

Day	Breakfast	Lunch	Dinner	Notes
Day 6	Egg Wraps with Sautéed Mushroom & Swiss Cheese (pg 37)	Nicoise Salad (pg 62)	Grilled Lamb Skewers with Cucumber-Yogurt Sauce (pg 79)	
Day 7	Protein "Fluff" with Chopped Nuts (pg 39)	Spicy Coconut Curry with Chicken & Cauliflower (pg 64)	Shrimp & Avocado Salad Stuffed Peppers (pg 45)	Focus on protein and healthy fats today. pen_spark

WEEK 2

Day	Breakfast	Lunch	Dinner	Notes
Day 8	Keto Frittata with Spinach, Mushrooms, & Goat Cheese (pg 25)	Shrimp & Avocado Salad Stuffed Peppers (pg 45)	Baked Cod with Lemon, Capers, & Olives (pg 73)	
Day 9	Shakshuka-Inspired Scramble with Italian Sausage (pg 31)	Zucchini Noodle Salad with Grilled Chicken (pg 47)	Steak & Roasted Veggie Bowl (pg 60)	
Day 10	Baked Eggs in Avocado with Salsa & Cotija Cheese (pg 29)	Nicoise Salad with Grilled Tuna Steaks (pg 62)	Creamy Mushroom & Spinach Stuffed Chicken (pg 87)	Consider a slightly higher carb intake today.
Day 11	Egg Wraps with Ham, Cheddar, & Spinach (pg 37)	Asian Turkey Lettuce Wraps with Water Chestnuts (pg 49)	One-Pan Sausage, Peppers, & Onion Skillet (pg 89)	
Day 12	Cloud Eggs with Bacon & Scallions (pg 23)	Tuna Salad with Cucumber "Crackers" (pg 55)	Spicy Shrimp Tacos with Avocado Salsa (Pg 75)	Focus on protein and healthy fats today.

| **Day 13** | Protein "Fluff" with Berries & Cinnamon (pg 39) | Roast Beef and Havarti Roll-Ups with Spicy Mustard (pg 57) | Grilled Lamb Skewers with Yogurt Sauce (pg 79) |
| **Day 14** | Crustless Quiche with Smoked Salmon & Dill (pg 27) | Mason Jar Salad with Salmon & Lemon Vinaigrette (pg 58) | Air Fryer Pork Chops with Parmesan Crust (pg 91) |

Day	Breakfast	Lunch	Dinner	Notes
Day 15	Shakshuka-Inspired Scramble with Spinach & Feta (pg 31)	Nicoise Salad with Smoked Salmon (pg 62)	Steak Salad w/ Blue Cheese & Balsamic (pg 51)	
Day 16	Protein "Fluff" with Cacao Nibs & Peanut Butter (pg 39)	Shrimp & Avocado Salad Stuffed Peppers (pg 45)	Tofu Scramble with Black Beans & Salsa (pg 95)	Focus on protein and healthy fats today.
Day 17	Cloud Eggs with Tomato, Basil, & Mozzarella (pg 23)	Mason Jar Salad with Salmon & Lemon Vinaigrette (pg 58)	Asian Turkey Lettuce Wraps with Kimchi (pg 49)	
Day 18	Keto Egg Bites with Bacon & Cheddar (pg 33)	Roast Beef and Havarti Roll-Ups with Dijon Mustard (pg 57)	Zucchini Noodle Salad with Grilled Chicken (pg 47)	Consider a slightly higher carb intake today.
Day 19	Crustless Broccoli, Mushroom & Swiss Quiche (pg 27)	Tuna Salad with Cucumber "Crackers" & Hot Sauce (pg55)	Air Fryer Pork Chops with Parmesan Crust (pg 91)	

Day 20	Egg Wraps with Sausage, Peppers, & Onions (pg 37)	Spicy Coconut Curry w/ Chicken & Cauliflower (pg 64)	Chicken Stuffed Poblano Peppers (pg 85)	Focus on whole-food carbs and healthy fats today.
Day 21	Baked Eggs in Avocado with Chorizo (pg 29)	Low-Carb Chicken Cobb Salad with Ranch Dressing (pg 53)	Scrambled Eggs with Smoked Salmon & Dill (pg 35) pen_spark	

CONCLUSION

Throughout this book, you've discovered the potential of the metabolic confusion diet tailored specifically for your endomorph body type. You've learned the science behind this approach, unlocked delicious and satisfying recipes, and experienced the structure of a 21-day meal plan. Now, it's time to apply this knowledge and make this plan your own.

This book is a starting point, not the final destination. Your metabolic confusion journey will evolve as you do. Be proud of taking this step toward better health, and continue learning, experimenting, and discovering the diet approach that empowers your endomorph body to thrive.

We'd love to hear how this book and the metabolic confusion plan have impacted your life. Please leave an honest review. Your feedback helps us improve future resources and inspires others on their own health journeys.

Thank you for being part of this exciting approach to nutrition and wellness!